HIGH COLLAGEN FOOD LIST

A COMPREHENSIVE GUIDE TO GLASSY SKIN, SUPPLE JOINTS, LUSH HAIR, STRONG NAILS, FAT LOSS AND DROPPING INCHES

JENNIE NUEL M.D.

Table of Contents

INTRODUCTION

The book "The High Collagen Food List: A Comprehensive Guide For Glassy Skin, Supple Joints, Lush Hair, Healthy Nails, Fat loss and Dropping Inches" is an exposé of the inherent benefits of a protein that we have paid little attention to! However, the quest for youthful vitality and classic beauty frequently returns us to one essential component: collagen.

The most prevalent protein in our bodies, collagen, is essential for maintaining healthy skin, bones, joints, and overall body function. Even so, a lot of us unintentionally overlook this vital protein in our diets.

This book is your guide to using a well-balanced diet to maximize the benefits of collagen. The collagen diet is a comprehensive approach to wellbeing that can change your life, whether your goal is to support your joints, brighten your skin, or just feel better overall.

We shall explore the science of collagen in the pages that follow, as well as how it affects your appearance and overall health. We will also find a plethora of foods high in collagen that can nourish your body from the inside out. This guide will help you on your path to optimal health by providing you with useful success suggestions and delicious recipes.

Thus, this book will help and motivate you at every stage of your journey, regardless of whether you are just starting out or want to expand on your knowledge. Prepare to set out on a life-changing adventure to become a healthier, more radiant version of yourself. The journey with collagen begins now!

CHAPTER ONE

UNDERSTANDING COLLAGEN

In the realm of health and beauty, collagen is more than just a catchphrase; it is the fundamental component that makes up our bodies' structural integrity. We shall study collagen in this chapter, including what it is, why it is important for our health, the many kinds of collagen, and how its functions affect our overall health.

What is collagen?

Collagen is a fibrous protein known as the main building block of connective tissues found all over the body. Frequently called the "glue" that binds our bodies together, it gives our skin, bones, muscles, tendons, and ligaments shape, sturdiness, and support. Collagen is actually one of the most prevalent proteins in the human body, accounting for around 30% of all proteins.

Think of collagen as the structural glue that binds tissues and cells together while enabling them to grow. Collagen's structural components are long chains of amino acids, mainly hydroxyproline, proline, and glycine, which are coiled into triple helices. Collagen possesses a distinct structure that contributes to its strength and durability.

Apart from its structural function, collagen is essential for wound healing, tissue repair, and preserving skin suppleness. The natural production of collagen in the body decreases with age, resulting in the appearance of wrinkles, drooping skin, and stiff joints. Consequently, in order to maintain general health and vigor, obtaining enough collagen from your food or supplements becomes more and more crucial.

Collagen is essential for overall health and well-being since it supports numerous physiological processes and is necessary for preserving the body's structural integrity.

Benefits of Collagen to the Body

Collagen is crucial for the following main reasons:

Structural Support: The skin, bones, tendons, ligaments, and muscles all rely on collagen to give them structural support. It creates a scaffold like network that provides resilience, flexibility, and strength to tissues so they can bear mechanical stress without losing their shape.

Skin Health: Collagen is essential for preserving the suppleness and integrity of the skin. It serves as the support system for the epidermis, the skin's outer layer, and forms the basis of the dermis, the skin's middle layer. Collagen fibers lessen the look of wrinkles and fine lines by keeping the skin moisturized, firm, and smooth.

Joint Function: A large part of cartilage, the pliable tissue that surrounds and cushions joints, is collagen. It facilitates painless and seamless joint movement by preserving the flexibility and integrity of cartilage. Collagen is essential for healthy joints because as we age, our collagen levels decrease and cause joint stiffness and discomfort.

Bone Strength: Collagen plays a vital role in the strength, suppleness, and resilience of bone tissue. It creates the framework for the deposition of minerals like calcium and phosphorus, giving structural support and averting osteoporosis and fractures.

Gut Health: Collagen supports the structure and functionality of the intestinal lining by aiding in the preservation of the gastrointestinal tract's integrity. This can enhance nutrition absorption and digestion while preventing the leaky gut syndrome.

Wound Healing: Collagen is essential for tissue repair and wound healing. It speeds up wound closure, encourages skin cell migration and proliferation, and aids in the formation of a scaffold for the creation of new tissue.

Hair and Nail Health: Collagen helps keep hair and nails strong and resilient by reducing the likelihood of brittleness, breaking, and splitting.

Getting enough collagen from your food or supplements can help you stay healthy, energetic, and live a long life.

Primary Collagen Types and Functions:

The family of proteins known as collagen is diverse, with different kinds of the protein fulfilling distinct roles in the body. The following are some of the primary forms of collagen and their purposes:

Type I Collagen: This is the most prevalent kind of collagen in the body. It is mostly present in the skin, bones, tendons, and teeth.

Function: It contributes to the integrity and stability of these tissues by giving them structural support, strength, and resilience. Type I collagen plays a vital role in the skin, helping to keep it hydrated, firm, and elastic while also minimizing wrinkles and enhancing the appearance of youthful skin.

Type II collagen|: This is mostly present in cartilage, the pliable tissue that surrounds and cushions joints.

Function: It gives cartilage structural stability and suppleness to ensure pain-free, seamless joint mobility. Type II collagen is essential for preserving joint health and averting diseases like osteoarthritis.

Type III collagen: This is is mostly present in blood vessels, the skin, and internal organs including the liver and lungs.

Function: It gives these tissues elasticity and structural support, which increases their tensile strength and durability. Type III collagen promotes cardiovascular health by preserving the suppleness and integrity of blood vessel walls.

Type IV Collagen: Plays a significant role in basement membranes, which control molecular transport between tissues and offer structural support. It serves to bind epithelial cells to underlying tissues, forming a network akin to a scaffold that promotes tissue architecture and function.

Function: Type IV collagen is necessary for the glomerular basement membrane's construction and operation, which is critical for blood pressure management and kidney filtration.

Type V Collagen: Mostly present in connective tissue, skin, and bone, type V collagen is a trace amount of the extracellular matrix.

Function: It contributes to the stability and structure of tissue by controlling the assembly and arrangement of collagen fibers. In the dermal layer of the skin, type V collagen contributes to the creation of fibrils and works in concert with other types of collagen to maintain the suppleness and strength of the skin.

Type VII Collagen: The specialized structures known as anchoring fibrils serve as a vital link between the dermis (the middle layer of skin) and the epidermis (the outer layer of skin).

Function: By attaching epidermal cells to the basement membrane and limiting the separation of skin layers, it aids in preserving the structural integrity of the skin.

Collagen Type X: This is mostly present in the growth plates of growing bones, where it is essential for cartilage mineralization and ossification.

Function: It controls the endochondral ossification process, which is the process by which bone replaces cartilage in the developing skeleton. Type X collagen plays a crucial role in bone remodeling and repair processes, especially in areas where bone growth or regeneration is occurring.

Even though these collagen types are less common than types I, II, and III, they are nonetheless necessary for the body's tissues and organs to retain their structural integrity, suppleness, and functionality.

Indices of Insufficient Collagen

Our bodies can create insufficient amounts of collagen or the collagen that does exist will deteriorate more quickly than new collagen can grow. This can result in a number of deficiencies, such as:

- Skin sagging and wrinkles
- Joint discomfort and stiffness
- Weakness and reduced muscle mass
- Hair and nail breakage
- Digestive problems

Factors that can deplete collagen in the body:

While aging may not be the only factor that is affecting the decline of collagen in your body, other factors to lookout for include:

- Sugar consumption
- Poor sleep
- Excessive consumption of soda
- Consumption of French fries and other fried foods
- Smoking
- Sun bathing
- Excessive alcohol intake
- Hormonal changes
- Chronic stress
- Lack of exercise
- Genetics
- Medical conditions such as rheumatoid arthritis, lupus
- Nutritional deficiencies like Vitamin C, E , and omega -3 fatty acid
- Environmental pollutants like exposure to heavy metals and toxins

The first step to maximizing the benefits of a collagen-rich diet comprehends the significance of collagen and its function in our bodies. We will look at ways to maximize your intake of collagen to support your health and beauty from the inside out.

CHAPTER 2

THE SCIENCE BEHIND COLLAGEN DIET

This chapter takes us on an exploration of the complex realm of the collagen diet, where nutrition and science come together to provide the keys to ultimate health and beauty. Because of its amazing qualities, collagen—often heralded as the secret to eternal youth—has drawn the interest of scientists and health enthusiasts alike.

We shall examine the benefits of collagen that research has proven, from its involvement in metabolism and weight management to its effects on skin renewal and anti-aging. Collagen is a key component of contemporary wellness.

We will also look at the most recent investigations and studies that provide insight into the significant impact of collagen on a range of human health issues. We will sort through the data to separate truth from fiction and explore the full potential of the collagen diet, from cutting-edge discoveries to clinical trials.

As we explore the complex linkages between collagen biology and nutrition, we shall arm ourselves with knowledge that has the potential to completely transform the way we think about health and appearance.

Collagen is essential for both health and beauty and has a lot of impact on our appearance and health, including:

Increased Skin Elasticity and Hydration: Research has shown that supplementing with collagen can greatly increase the elasticity and hydration of the skin. In the Journal of Cosmetic Dermatology, for instance, a study's findings after eight weeks of collagen supplementation revealed a noteworthy improvement in skin hydration and a decrease in wrinkle depth when compared to the placebo group.

Reduction of Inflammation and Joint Pain: Studies indicate that collagen supplements may help reduce inflammation and joint pain brought on by diseases like osteoarthritis. The journal Seminars in Arthritis and Rheumatism published a meta-analysis that indicated collagen supplementation was useful in lowering pain and enhancing physical function in osteoarthritis patients.

Support for Bone Health: Research has demonstrated the critical role collagen plays in maintaining bone health, with supplements boosting bone mineral density and lowering fracture risk. According to a research in the Journal of Medicinal Food, postmenopausal women who took collagen supplements for a full year saw a notable improvement in bone mineral density in comparison to the group that received a placebo.

Accelerated development of Hair and Nails: According to preliminary study, collagen supplements may improve the health of hair and nails by encouraging stronger and faster development. Although further research is required to validate these effects, preliminary research and anecdotal data are encouraging.

Weight management: Collagen has been shown to help in maintaining lean muscle mass and encouraging satiety. Further research is necessary to completely understand the benefits of collagen supplementation on appetite suppression and muscle loss prevention during calorie restriction.

CHAPTER 3

GETTING STARTED WITH THE COLLAGEN DIET

Starting a collagen diet is a powerful step toward improving your appearance from the inside out and reaching your full potential. We will walk you through the collagen diet's initial steps in this chapter, providing you with useful pointers, doable recommendations, and customized plans to ensure your success.

Evaluating Your Existing Lifestyle and Diet

Assessing your current dietary practices and lifestyle factors is crucial before beginning the collagen diet. Evaluating your food consumption, exercise regimen, sleep habits, stress levels, and general state of well-being can give you important information about what you are doing well and what still needs improvement. This self-evaluation forms the basis for establishing reasonable objectives and designing a customized plan that suits your unique requirements and preferences.

Having Reasonable Objectives

Establishing attainable goals is essential to sustaining motivation and adhering to your collagen diet plan. Whether your aims are to manage weight, promote joint function, improve overall well-being, or improve skin health, it is critical to set precise, quantifiable goals that are doable. To keep motivated and focused on your journey, break down larger goals into smaller, manageable tasks, recognize, and celebrate your accomplishments along the way.

Organizing Your Snacks and Meals

Organizing and preparing meals is crucial to following the collagen diet successfully. Make sure to include a range of collagen-rich foods in your meal and snack plans, including leafy greens, berries, nuts, chicken, fish, and bone broth. To keep things interesting and pleasurable, try out different recipes and meal ideas. You may also think about batch cooking or meal preparation to save time and organize your schedule.

Advice for a Successful Collagen Diet Introduction

Making the switch to a collagen diet can be a fulfilling and thrilling path to better health and appearance. Here are some helpful hints to get you started on the right track with this dietary adjustment:

1. Get Started Gradually: Allow your taste buds and digestive system time to adjust while gradually incorporating foods and supplements high in collagen into your diet. Start by adding modest portions of foods high in collagen, such as leafy greens, berries, almonds, chicken, fish, and bone broth, to your meals and snacks. You can progressively increase your intake of these foods over time, as you get more acclimated to them.

2. Remain Consistent: Observing the collagen diet consistently is essential to getting results. Make it a habit to include foods high in collagen in your daily meals and snacks. Remain true to your strategy even when faced with temptations or on hectic days. To help you remain on track and incorporate collagen consumption into your routine, set reminders or establish a food plan.

3. Drink Plenty of Water: Skin health and collagen formation depend on adequate hydration. To keep your skin moisturized and encourage the formation of collagen in your skin, make sure you drink lots of water throughout the day. Try to consume 8 to 10 glasses of water a day, and think about including foods high in water content, such as citrus fruits, cucumbers, and watermelon, in your diet.

4. Combine Collagen with Vitamin C: To optimize absorption and efficacy, combine collagen-rich foods with sources of vitamin C, as vitamin C is necessary for the synthesis of collagen. Add foods like broccoli, bell peppers, kiwi, strawberries, and citrus fruits to your meals to make sure you are getting enough vitamin C to boost the creation of collagen.

5. Listen to Your Body: Keep an eye on how the collagen diet affects your body and adjust as necessary. Since each person has different dietary requirements and tolerances, pay attention to your body's signals and modify your strategy as necessary. Seek advice from a healthcare provider if you encounter any bad reactions or gastrointestinal distress.

6. Experiment with dishes: Try out different dishes and meal ideas to keep your collagen-rich meals engaging and pleasurable. To keep things interesting in the kitchen, get creative and experiment with various cooking techniques, flavor combinations, and culinary methods. Search our recipe book for collagen-friendly recipes, and feel free to modify them to suit your tastes.

7. Make a Plan: Making a plan for your meals and snacks in advance can help you stick to the collagen diet and prevent you from reaching for bad choices when you are hungry. Make a grocery list, plan your meals, and prepare your items in advance once a week. To save time and guarantee that collagen-rich foods are always available, think about bulk cooking or meal preparing.

8. Remain Upbeat and Patient: Keep in mind that things do not always happen right away and that growth takes time. Remain optimistic, patient, and dedicated to your collagen journey, understanding that each healthy decision you make will get you closer to your desired appearance and overall well-being. No matter how minor your victories may have been along the road, acknowledge them and keep pushing forward with self-assurance and resolve.

Overcoming Typical Obstacles

The collagen diet has many advantages for both health and appearance, but there are drawbacks as well. Here are some typical roadblocks you could run into while on the collagen diet, along with solutions:

1. Social Contexts:

Challenge: Food and beverages that may not be in line with the collagen diet are frequently the focal point of social engagements and gatherings. When friends or family tempt you, it can be difficult to stay true to your goal.
Method: To prevent cravings, consume a meal or snack high in collagen before going to social activities. Offer to share your own collagen-friendly food, or graciously turn down anything that does not align with your diet. Instead of obsessing on the meal, concentrate on enjoying the company and the conversation.

2. Wants:

The collagen diet can be challenging to stick to because sugary or processed food cravings can strike at any time, especially during stressful or boring times.
Plan: Find healthier ways to sate your desires, including fresh fruit, protein-rich snacks, or smoothies with collagen included. When cravings arise, use mindfulness exercises to tune into your body's signals of hunger and fullness and use activities like walking, reading, or a hobby to divert your attention.

3. Time Restrictions:

Problem: Scheduling meals, preparing them, and consuming collagen can be difficult when there are time restraints and hectic schedules.

Strategy: Set aside specific time each week to organize your meals, shop for groceries, and prepare ingredients. This will help you make meal planning and preparation a priority. Look out for quick and simple meals that are high in collagen and can be made in advance such as salads, stir-fries, or smoothies. To speed up the process, think about spending money on meal delivery services or timesaving kitchen appliances.

4. Preferences for Taste:

Challenge: It may be difficult for some people to include foods high in collagen in their diet due to their unattractive texture or taste.
Strategy: Try a variety of cooking techniques, flavor combos, and recipe formulations to discover collagen-rich meals that you enjoy. Use your creativity in the kitchen to include collagen powder into beverages, baked goods, stews, and soups to offer an extra nutritional punch without drastically changing the flavor.

5. Travel and Eating Out:

Challenge: Because there may be fewer or unfamiliar options when traveling or dining out, adhering to the collagen diet may be difficult.
Strategy: Plan ahead by looking into collagen-friendly accommodations at your visit or selecting eateries with a menu that is full of flexible, healthful options. When traveling, have collagen snacks or supplements with you, and do not be hesitant to ask restaurant personnel to modify or substitute ingredients to suit your dietary requirements.

6. Diet plateau:

Challenge: On every diet, you may encounter setbacks or plateaus where you lose ground or shortly stray from your intended path.
Strategy: Remain committed to your long-term objectives and keep in mind that obstacles are a normal part of the process.

CHAPTER 4

COLLAGEN RICH FOODS

We explore the wide range of collagen-rich foods that form the basis of the collagen diet in this chapter. Not only do these nutrient-dense alternatives taste great, but they also give your body the fundamental building blocks it needs to boost the production of collagen, promote skin health, and improve overall wellbeing. Let us examine the vast array of collagen-rich meals at your disposal:

25 collagen sources derived from animals:

1.Bone Broth:

Simmering animal bones (such as chicken, cattle, or fish) with vegetables, herbs, and spices in water for a long time results in rich bone broth, which is highly nourishing. The simmering process releases the collagen and gelatin from the bones, making a tasty and nutrient-rich broth. It is possible to use bone broth as a base for soups, stews, sauces, and other foods, or to enjoy it on its own as a warm and pleasant beverage. Frequent use of bone broth can offer a concentrated amount of minerals, amino acids, and collagen to maintain the health of your skin, joints, and bones.

2. Chicken Cartilage and Skin:

Collagen-rich chicken skin and cartilage are especially beneficial when slow-cooked or boiled in soups and stews. A large portion of the collagen in chicken skin gives the meat's texture and flavor when cooked. Collagen is plentiful in cartilage, which is found in joints and connective tissues. You can get natural collagen and critical amino acids required for collagen formation by including chicken skin and cartilage in your meals.

3. Connective Tissues from Beef:

Shank, oxtail, and brisket are among the beef cuts with connective tissues that are great providers of collagen. Collagen-rich connective tissues, such as tendons, ligaments, and fascia, become soft and delicious when cooked gently. These cuts of beef make tasty and collagen-rich meals like pot roast, beef stew, and braised beef. Incorporating cow connective tissues into your diet can improve the health of your skin, joints, and bones while also giving your food a richer taste.

4. Fish bones and skin:

Collagen is present in the skin and bones of fatty fish, such as salmon, mackerel, and sardines. Fish collagen has a comparable molecular structure to human skin and tissues, making it highly accessible and easily absorbed. You can get a natural supply of collagen and omega-3 fatty acids by eating fish that still has the skin and bones on it or by making soups and stews with fish broth. Fish collagen is a nutrient-dense complement to any diet that promotes bone, joint, and skin health.

5. Pork Cut Off:

Another natural source of collagen is pork skin, which also contains gelatin. Crispy pigskin—also referred to as pork rinds or chicharrones—is a widely consumed food in many global cultures. By adding tasty and collagen-rich pork skin to your meals, you may enhance the health of your skin, joints, and bones.

6. Gelatin Rich Foods:

The process of boiling animal skin, tendons, ligaments, and bones yields gelatin, a protein rich in collagen. Gelatin-containing foods offer a concentrated dose of collagen and gelatin. Examples of these foods include gelatin desserts, marshmallows, gummy sweets, and some dairy products including yogurt and cream cheese. You can give your skin, joints, and bones extra support by including these foods in your diet.

7. Eggs:

Protein known as collagen type I, which is present in egg whites, is comparable to the collagen present in human skin and bones. Although not as high in collagen as other animal products, eggs still contain all the key amino acids needed to synthesize collagen. Eggs are a good source of minerals and protein for maintaining the general health of your skin and tissues.

8. Goose and Duck:

Ducks and geese, as well as other poultry, have skin and connective tissues that are rich in collagen. To release collagen and produce tasty dishes, these meats can be slow-cooked, braised, or roasted. In particular, skin from ducks and geese can be rendered to make duck fat, a tasty cooking fat that can be utilized in a variety of culinary applications. You can enhance the health of your skin, joints, and bones by consuming duck and goose as extra sources of collagen in your diet.

9. Shellfish:

Collagen is a component of the connective tissues and shells of shellfish, including shrimp, crab, lobster, and mussels. You can get a natural supply of collagen and minerals by eating shellfish whole or by making broth from the shells. Easy to digest, shellfish collagen can promote bone, joint, and skin health while enhancing the flavor of your food.

10. Organ Meats:

Organ meats, such as those from the liver, heart, kidney, and tongue, are high in nutrients and contain connective tissues that are high in collagen. Organ meats are highly valued in many cultures for their culinary diversity and health benefits, despite being less popular in Western diets. Cooking organ meats in a variety of ways, like sautéing, roasting, or braising, can extract collagen and produce tasty meals. You can get a concentrated supply of collagen and other key nutrients to support overall health and vigor by including organ meats in your diet.

11. Chicken Feet:

Gelatin and collagen are abundant in poultry feet, including those of chickens and turkeys. Connective tissues, like cartilage and tendons of birds, have high concentrations of collagen. You may use poultry feet to make a rich, savory broth that is full of nutrients, or you can use them in soups, stews, and braises to add texture and extract collagen.

12. Bone Marrow:
Collagen, lipids, and other nutrients are abundant in bone marrow, which is located in the interior of bones. Slow cooking or roasting of the bones causes the fat and collagen in the marrow to melt and form a rich, tasty gelatin. Spreading bone marrow over toast, adding it to soups and stews for more flavor, or using it as a cooking oil to roast meats or vegetables are all delicious uses for it.

13. Hocks of pork:
Pig hocks, sometimes referred to as pig knuckles or pork trotters, are meat portions that are heavy in collagen-rich connective tissues. Pork hocks that are slow-cooked will have more collagen broken down and have a richer, more delicious flesh with lots of gelatin. Traditional recipes including soups, stews, and braises frequently use pork hocks because they enhance the dish's richness and depth of flavor.

14. Meat Cuts with Bones:
Meats with visible bones, such oxtails, shanks, and ribs, have connective tissues that are rich in collagen. These beef slices absorb more taste and richness from the slow cooking process, which breaks down the collagen. Bone-in meat pieces add flavor and texture to a range of recipes, such as braises roasts, stews, and soups.

15. Pork Belly:
Pork belly is a high-fat pork cut that has layers of skin and fat rich in collagen. Pork belly becomes a soft, luscious texture, thanks to the breakdown of collagen during slow cooking. Pork belly lends richness and taste to a variety of dishes, including braised pork belly, crispy pork belly, and pork belly ramen.

16. Tendons of beef:
Rich in collagen, beef tendons are fibrous, strong fibers that join muscles to bones. Beef tendons can develop a soft, gelatinous texture when boiled slowly leading to more collagen breakdown. Asian cooking frequently uses cow tendons, especially in soups and braises where they provide the food with flavor and texture.

17. Tripe made with beef:
The edible stomach lining of cattle is known as beef tripe, and it is a great source of collagen and other minerals. Tripe is a common ingredient in many traditional soups, stews, and curries found all over the world. Cooking beef tripe slowly helps produce a tasty and filling dish by tenderizing the collagen-rich tissue.

18. Concentrate Bone Broth:
Making bone broth concentrate involves boiling bones and connective tissues in water, then reducing the liquid to get a concentrated broth. Bone broth concentrate is a condensed version of bone broth. You can add bone broth concentrate straight to soups, stews, sauces, and other foods, or you can reconstituted it with water to enhance the flavor and nutritional value.

19. Giblets of chicken:
The term "chicken giblets" describes the edible internal organs of fowl, such as the neck, gizzard, liver, and heart. These organs are versatile and full of nutrients and collagen. You may make tasty recipes like giblet gravy, pâté, or stuffing out of chicken giblets by sautéing, roasting, or simmering them.

20. Pork Cracklings with Skin:
Pork skin cracklings are crispy appetizers produced from fried pork skin, sometimes referred to as pork rinds or cracklings. You can eat pork skin cracklings as a snack on their own or as a garnish for casseroles, soups, and salads. They are high in fat and collagen. They give a healthy dose of collagen-rich nutrients to meals while giving them a crunchy texture and savory flavor.

21. Goat or Lamb:

Shank, shoulder, and neck slices of lamb and goat are high in collagen, just like those of beef. Slow cooking, breaks down the collagen in these cuts and produce dishes that are tender and tasty. Roasts, braises, and stews made from lamb or goat are common ways to eat these meats and reap the benefits of their high collagen content.

22. Chicken Bones:

Ducks and geese, in addition to chicken and turkey, also produce bones that are high in collagen. You may make a filling, nutrient- and collagen-rich poultry broth by slowly boiling chicken bones with spices and vegetables. You can enjoy poultry bone broth on its own as a nutritious drink or use it as a base for soups, sauces, and risottos.

23. Bone Marrow Soup:

Rich in collagen, lipids, and other nutrients, bone marrow is located in the core of big bones. A tasty bone marrow broth can be made by roasting the bone marrow and then boiling it with water and spices. As a stand-alone dish or as a foundation for soups and stews, bone marrow broth has a strong umami taste and is rich and flavorful.

24. Roe of Fish:

Omega-3 fatty acids and collagen are abundant in fish roe, commonly referred to as fish eggs or caviar. Eating fish roe offers a concentrated form of collagen and other vital nutrients that help maintain the health of your skin, joints, and bones. You can eat fish roe as a delicacy on its own or as a garnish for salads, sushi, and other foods.

25. Liver of beef:

Rich in vitamins, minerals, collagen, and other vital nutrients, beef liver is an organ meat that is high in nutrition. Although connective tissues have a higher collagen content, cow liver nevertheless offers a range of nutrients that promote general health and vigor. Improved skin, joint, and bone health are just a few of the health advantages of having cow liver in your diet.

There are many ways to include foods high in collagen in your diet, and these animal-based collagen sources provide a variety of alternatives. There are many delectable and nourishing options to support skin, joint, and bone health, regardless of your preference for beef liver, fish roe, chicken bone broth, or goat stew.

30 plant-based nutritional sources

1. Greens with leaves:
Rich in vitamins and minerals, leafy greens including spinach, kale, Swiss chard, and collard greens promote the production of collagen. These greens are rich in vitamin K, which promotes bone health, and vitamin C, which is necessary for the synthesis of collagen. Consuming leafy greens can supply a range of nutrients that promote the general health of your skin, joints, and bones.

2. Bell Peppers:
Bell peppers, especially the red and yellow kinds, are a great way to get vitamin C, which is necessary for the synthesis of collagen. Vitamin C is essential for keeping healthy skin, joints, and bones since it is critical in the conversion of proline and lysine into collagen. Bell peppers are a nutrient-dense food that can boost collagen production and improve general health and vigor.

3. Berries:
Antioxidants, vitamins, and minerals included in berries such as strawberries, raspberries, blueberries, and blackberries help to support the synthesis of collagen. These fruits are rich in vitamin C, which encourages the formation of new collagen and helps shield it from oxidative stress-related damage. A tasty and nourishing strategy to promote bone, joint, and skin health is by including berries in your diet.

4. Citrus Fruits:

Vitamin C is abundant in citrus fruits, including oranges, lemons, limes, and grapefruits. Vitamin C is necessary for the manufacture of collagen. Vitamin C is essential for the synthesis of collagen, which supports and preserves the integrity of the skin, joints, and bones. Citrus fruits are a nutrient-dense and refreshing method to enhance general health and vitality in your diet.

5. Tomatoes:

Tomatoes are a great source of lycopene, a potent antioxidant that helps shield collagen from harm from free radicals. By lowering the danger of UV damage and early aging, lycopene also promotes the health of the skin. Tomatoes are a tasty and nutrient-dense strategy to encourage the development of collagen and maintain healthy skin, joints, and bones.

6. Avocado:

Avocados are a fruit high in nutrients, full of vitamins, minerals, and good fats that promote the production of collagen. Avocados are rich in vitamin E, an antioxidant that helps shield collagen from oxidative stress-related damage. A diet rich in avocados can supply vital nutrients that promote bone, joint, and skin health.

7. Soy-Based Products:

Protein and amino acids found in soy products like edamame, tempeh, and tofu aid in the formation of collagen. Genistein, which is abundant in soy, has been demonstrated to increase the release of collagen and enhance skin suppleness. You may get plant-based forms of protein and nutrients that promote the general health of your skin and tissues by including soy products in your diet.

8. Seeds and Nuts:

Nuts and seeds are high in protein, good fats, vitamins, and minerals that promote collagen synthesis including almonds, walnuts, flaxseeds, and chia seeds. These foods contain amino acids that are necessary for the synthesis of collagen, such as proline and lysine. You can obtain a range of nutrients that promote bone, joint, and skin health by including nuts and seeds in your diet.

9. Legumes:

Excellent providers of protein, fiber, vitamins, and minerals that aid in the manufacture of collagen including legumes, such as beans, lentils, and chickpeas. These foods include amino acids that are necessary for the synthesis of collagen, such as proline and lysine. Legumes are a plant-based source of minerals and protein that can help maintain the general health of your skin and tissues.

10. Spirulina

Rich in protein, vitamins, minerals, and antioxidants, spirulina is an alga that is high in nutrients that promotes the synthesis of collagen. Glycine and proline, two amino acids found in spirulina, are necessary for the synthesis of collagen. You may get plant-based protein and nutrients that promote the health of your skin, joints, and bones by including spirulina in your diet.

11. Seeds:

Hemp, sunflower, and pumpkin seeds are a few examples of seeds that are high in protein, good fats, vitamins, and minerals that promote the production of collagen. Particularly high in zinc and copper, these seeds are vital cofactors for the synthesis of collagen. You can obtain a range of nutrients that promote bone, joint, and skin health by including seeds in your diet.

12. Beans:

Beans that are high in protein, fiber, vitamins, and minerals that promote collagen formation including kidney, pinto, and black beans. These legumes are rich in amino acids, such as lysine and proline, which are necessary for the synthesis of collagen. You can get plant-based protein and nutrients that promote the health of your skin and tissues by including beans in your diet.

13. Quinoa:

Quinoa is high in fiber, protein, and vitamins and minerals that aid in the production of collagen. Proline and lysine, two amino acids required for the synthesis of collagen, are among the nine essential amino acids found in quinoa. You may get plant-based protein and nutrients that promote the health of your skin, joints, and bones by including quinoa in your diet.

14. Soy:

Rich in protein, vitamins, minerals, and antioxidants that promote collagen formation, soybeans are a very adaptable legume. Genistein, a substance found in soybeans, has been shown to increase collagen synthesis and enhance skin suppleness. You can obtain plant-based protein and nutrients that promote the general health of your skin and tissues by including soybeans in your diet.

15. Buckwheat:

Rich in protein, fiber, vitamins, and minerals that promote collagen formation, buckwheat is a gluten-free grain. Buckwheat is a good source of rutin, an antioxidant flavonoid that helps shield collagen from oxidative stress-related damage. Buckwheat is a plant-based source of protein and nutrients that are beneficial to the health of your skin, joints, and bones.

16. Chia Seeds:

Chia seeds are little seeds that are rich in fiber, protein, and other nutrients that help to promote the production of collagen. Omega-3 fatty acids, which support healthy skin and help prevent inflammation, are especially abundant in chia seeds. Chia seeds are a plant-based source of minerals and protein that can help maintain the general health of your skin and tissues.

17. Algae:

Spirulina and chlorella are two examples of algae that are high in protein, vitamins, minerals, and antioxidants that aid in the creation of collagen. These algae are rich in amino acids, such as proline and glycine, which are necessary for the synthesis of collagen. Algae are plant-based sources of protein and nutrients that are beneficial to the health of your skin, joints, and bones.

18. Seeds from sesame plants:

These seeds are rich in protein, good fats, vitamins, and minerals that aid in the formation of collagen. The minerals manganese, copper, and zinc found in sesame seeds are necessary cofactors for the synthesis of collagen. Sesame seeds are a plant-based source of minerals and protein that can help maintain the general health of your skin and tissues.

19. Sweet potatoes:

Sweet potatoes are a wholesome root vegetable that are high in antioxidants, vitamins, and minerals that promote the production of collagen. Beta-carotene, which helps shield collagen from oxidative stress damage, is especially abundant in sweet potatoes. Sweet potatoes are a plant-based source of nutrients that promote bone, joint, and skin health. Include them in your diet.

20. Grains of Brown Rice:

Whole grains like brown rice are high in fiber, protein, and other nutrients that promote the production of collagen. Gamma-oryzanol, a substance found in brown rice, helps shield collagen from oxidative damage brought on by free radicals. You may get plant-based forms of nutrients that promote the general health of your skin and tissues by including brown rice in your diet.

21. Flaxseeds:

Flaxseeds are high in fiber, chemicals with antioxidant qualities called lignans, and omega-3 fatty acids. Omega-3 fatty acids aid in the reduction of inflammation, and lignans may shield collagen. You may add flaxseeds to smoothies, cereal, or baked goods to add important nutrients that support bone, joint, and skin health to your diet.

22. Seeds from pumpkins:

Pulses, or pepitas, are seeds from pumpkins that are rich in fiber, protein, and a variety of vitamins and minerals. They are especially high in zinc, which is essential for the production of collagen and the healing of wounds. Savor pumpkin seeds on their own as a snack or add them to salads, yoghurt, or oatmeal for a nutritional boost.

23. Wheat germ:
The nutrient-rich embryo of the wheat kernel, known as wheat germ, is a concentrated source of antioxidants, vitamins, and minerals. It has vitamin E, an antioxidant that helps shield collagen from free radicals. To enhance the health of your skin, joints, and bones, sprinkle some wheat germ on your cereal, yogurt, or salads.

24. Brussels Sprouts:
Brussels sprouts are cruciferous vegetables that are high in antioxidants, fiber, vitamin C, and vitamin K. While vitamin K promotes bone health and mineralization, vitamin C is necessary for the creation of collagen. Brussels sprouts can be sautéed or roasted with garlic and olive oil to create a tasty and nourishing side dish that promotes general health and vigor.

25. Cabbage:
Green, crimson, and purple are just a few of the vibrant hues of this adaptable vegetable. Rich in fiber, antioxidants, and vitamin C, it promotes collagen formation and guards against oxidative stress. For an added nutritional and flavor boost, try cabbage raw in salads, fermented as sauerkraut, or cooked in stir-fries and soups.

26. Almonds:
Nutrient-dense almonds are high in fiber, protein, good fats, vitamin E, and other minerals. As an antioxidant, vitamin E aids in preventing free radical damage to collagen. For a tasty and nutrient-dense boost, you may eat almonds as a snack or add them to salads, smoothies, and homemade granola.

27. Oatmeal
Oats are whole grains that are high in fiber, protein, and other vitamins and

minerals, such as copper and zinc. These minerals are necessary cofactors for the manufacture of collagen, which maintains the health of the skin, joints, and bones. A substantial dish of oats topped with fruits, nuts, and seeds is a filling breakfast that helps you feel better all round.

28. Asparagus:
This is a nutrient dense vegetable rich in vitamins C, K, folate, and antioxidants. While vitamin K supports calcium absorption and bone health, vitamin C aids in the creation of collagen. Savor asparagus as an appetizer (steamed, roasted, or grilled), or add it to salads, omelets, or pasta dishes to boost their nutritional value and flavor.

29. Mushrooms:
When exposed to sunshine, mushrooms present a special plant-based source of vitamin D. Vitamin D indirectly promotes collagen synthesis and is essential for bone health and calcium absorption. To increase your intake of vitamin D and promote general health, include a variety of mushrooms in your meals, such as shiitake, portobello, and oyster mushrooms.

30. Broccoli:
Broccoli is a cruciferous vegetable that is high in antioxidants, fiber, vitamin K, and C. While vitamin K promotes bone health and density, vitamin C is necessary for the synthesis of collagen. Incorporate broccoli's nutritious advantages into your diet by steaming it as a side dish or adding it to stir-fries, salads, and soups.

By including these nutrient-rich plant-based sources in your diet, you may boost general health and vitality as well as supply the necessary building blocks for collagen formation. There are many tasty and nourishing options to pick from to increase your intake of collagen and support wellness from the inside out, irrespective of your preference for seeds, nuts, vegetables, or whole grains.

CHAPTER 5

CREATING COLLAGEN BOOSTING MEALS

Creating meals that not only entice your taste buds but also nourish your body from the inside out is what we call a culinary adventure. In this chapter, we explore the skill of blending nutrient-dense meals with collagen-rich components to make tasty dishes that support skin health, encourage collagen synthesis, and enhance overall wellbeing.

You will learn about the abundance of ingredients and their versatility that you can use to create a wide variety of dishes as we go deeper into the realm of collagen-boosting meals. Every element in your diet—from colorful fruits and vegetables to lean proteins, healthy fats, and whole grains—plays a crucial part in giving your body the nourishment it needs to create collagen and stay in maximum health.

With a wide range of recipes to suit every taste and dietary requirement, this chapter has you covered whether you are looking for ideas for a filling brunch, a tasty lunch, or a tasty dinner. As you set off on your collagen-boosting culinary journey, there is something for everyone to enjoy, from filling salads and rich soups to substantial main courses and indulgent desserts.

This chapter will give you useful advice, recipe ideas, and cooking methods to help you get the most out of collagen-rich foods and optimize their health benefits. You will discover how to maximize the benefits of collagen in every meal you make, whether you are cooking for your loved ones, yourself, or both. This will leave you feeling invigorated, renewed, and radiant from the inside out.

So grab your apron, sharpen your knives, and get ready to take part in a culinary adventure that highlights the beauty of dishes that promote collagen production. You will support the health of your skin, fuel your body, and experience the joy of eating clean, delicious food with every recipe you attempt and every meal you enjoy. Together, we can unleash the transforming potential of collagen in your kitchen and take your cuisine to new heights.

30 DAYS OF NUTRITIOUS BREAKFAST OPTIONS:

Day 1: Collagen Smoothie Bowl

Cooking Time: 5 minutes

Calories: 300-400

Blend together spinach, banana, almond milk, collagen powder, and your favorite berries. Top with granola, sliced fruit, and a drizzle of honey for a nutritious and delicious start to your day.

Day 2: Scrambled Eggs with Spinach and Tomatoes

Cooking Time: 10 minutes

Calories: 250-300

Whisk together eggs and cook with spinach and diced tomatoes. Serve with whole grain toast or avocado slices for a protein-packed breakfast that's rich in vitamins and minerals.

Day 3: Greek Yogurt Parfait with Berries and Almonds

Preparation Time: 5 minutes

Calories: 300-350

Layer Greek yogurt with fresh berries, almonds, and a sprinkle of granola for a creamy and satisfying breakfast that is high in protein, fiber, and antioxidants.

Day 4: Oatmeal with Sliced Banana and Almond Butter

Cooking Time: 10 minutes

Calories: 300-400

Cook rolled oats with almond milk and top with sliced banana, a dollop of almond butter, and a sprinkle of cinnamon for a warm and comforting breakfast that is full of fiber and healthy fats.

Day 5: Smoked Salmon and Avocado Toast

Preparation Time: 5 minutes

Calories: 350-400

Spread mashed avocado on whole grain toast and top with smoked salmon, sliced cucumber, and a squeeze of lemon juice for a savory and nutritious breakfast that is rich in omega-3 fatty acids.

Day 6: Collagen-Infused Pancakes with Maple Syrup

Cooking Time: 15 minutes

Calories: 300-350

Add collagen powder to your favorite pancake recipe and serve with maple syrup, fresh fruit, and a dollop of Greek yogurt for a fluffy and indulgent breakfast that supports collagen production.

Day 7: Chia Seed Pudding with Coconut Milk and Mango

Preparation Time: 5 minutes (+overnight)

Calories: 250-300

Mix chia seeds with coconut milk and let sit overnight. Top with diced mango, shredded coconut, and a sprinkle of hemp seeds for a creamy and tropical breakfast that is packed with omega-3s and fiber.

Day 8: Breakfast Burrito with Eggs, Black Beans, and Salsa

Cooking Time: 15 minutes

Calories: 350-400

Scramble eggs with black beans, diced bell peppers, and onions. Wrap in a whole grain tortilla and top with salsa, avocado, and a sprinkle of cheese for a hearty and flavorful breakfast that's perfect for on-the-go.

Day 9: Spinach and Feta Frittata

Cooking Time: 20 minutes

Calories: 300-350

Whisk together eggs with sautéed spinach, crumbled feta cheese, and cherry tomatoes. Bake until set and golden brown for a protein-rich breakfast that is perfect for feeding a crowd or meal prepping for the week.

Day 10: Acai Bowl with Granola and Mixed Berries

Preparation Time: 10 minutes

Calories: 350-450

Blend frozen acai with banana, almond milk, and spinach until smooth. Top with granola, mixed berries, sliced banana, and a drizzle of honey for a refreshing and antioxidant-rich breakfast that is bursting with flavor.

Day 11: Quinoa Breakfast Bowl with Roasted Vegetables

Cooking Time: 20 minutes

Calories: 350-400

Cook quinoa and serve with roasted vegetables, such as sweet potatoes, Brussels sprouts, and cherry tomatoes. Top with a fried egg and avocado slices for a hearty and nutritious breakfast that is loaded with fiber and protein.

Day 12: Cottage Cheese with Pineapple and Toasted Coconut

Preparation Time: 5 minutes

Calories: 250-300

Serve cottage cheese with diced pineapple, toasted coconut flakes, and a sprinkle of cinnamon for a creamy and tropical breakfast that is high in protein and calcium.

Day 13: Collagen-Boosting Smoothie with Kale, Pineapple, and Ginger

Preparation Time: 5 minutes

Calories: 250-300

Blend kale, pineapple, ginger, collagen powder, and coconut water until smooth. Serve with a slice of lemon for a refreshing and immune-boosting breakfast that is packed with vitamins and minerals.

Day 14: Whole Grain Toast with Peanut Butter and Sliced Apple

Preparation Time: 5 minutes

Calories: 300-350

Spread whole grain toast with peanut butter and top with thinly sliced apple and a sprinkle of cinnamon for a crunchy and satisfying breakfast that is rich in fiber and protein.

Day 15: Avocado and Tomato Breakfast Sandwich on Whole Grain Bread

Preparation Time: 10 minutes

Calories: 350-400

Layer mashed avocado and sliced tomato on whole grain bread. Top with a fried egg and a drizzle of hot sauce for a savory and nutrient-dense breakfast that is perfect for any time of day.

Day 16: Blueberry Chia Seed Muffins

Cooking Time: 25 minutes

Calories: 150-200 (per muffin)

Bake homemade blueberry chia seed muffins using whole-wheat flour, Greek yogurt, and fresh blueberries for a portable and delicious breakfast option that is high in fiber and antioxidants.

Day 17: Overnight Oats with Almond Milk, Chia Seeds, and Berries

Preparation Time: 5 minutes (+overnight)

Calories: 300-350

Mix rolled oats with almond milk, chia seeds, and your favorite berries. Let sit overnight in the refrigerator and top with sliced almonds and a drizzle of honey for a convenient and nutritious breakfast that is ready to enjoy in the morning.

Day 18: Veggie and Cheese Omelette

Cooking Time: 10 minutes

Calories: 300-350

Whisk together eggs and cook with sautéed bell peppers, onions, and spinach. Top with shredded cheese and fold in half for a protein-packed breakfast that is bursting with flavor and color.

Day 19: Coconut Flour Pancakes with Fresh Berries

Cooking Time: 15 minutes

Calories: 250-300

Make homemade coconut flour pancakes and serve with fresh berries, Greek yogurt, and a drizzle of maple syrup for a fluffy and gluten-free breakfast option that is rich in fiber and antioxidants.

Day 20: Breakfast Tacos with Scrambled Eggs, Black Beans, and Avocado

Cooking Time: 15 minutes

Calories: 350-400

Fill whole grain tortillas with scrambled eggs, black beans, diced avocado, and salsa for a hearty and satisfying breakfast that's perfect for taco Tuesday or any day of the week.

Day 21: Green Smoothie with Collagen Powder, Spinach, and Kiwi

Preparation Time: 5 minutes

Calories: 250-300

Blend spinach, kiwi, collagen powder, and coconut water until smooth. Serve with a sprinkle of chia seeds for a refreshing and nutrient-packed breakfast that is perfect for fueling your day.

Day 22: Breakfast Quinoa Bowl with Pecans and Maple Syrup

Cooking Time: 20 minutes

Calories: 300-350

Cook quinoa and serve with toasted pecans, sliced banana, and a drizzle of maple syrup for a warm and comforting breakfast that is high in protein and fiber.

Day 23: Greek Yogurt with Honey and Walnuts

Preparation Time: 5 minutes

Calories: 250-300

Serve Greek yogurt with a drizzle of honey and chopped walnuts for a creamy and satisfying breakfast that is rich in protein, probiotics, and healthy fats.

Day 24: Whole Grain Waffles with Greek Yogurt and Strawberries

Cooking Time: 15 minutes

Calories: 300-350

Make homemade whole grain waffles, serve with Greek yogurt, and sliced strawberries for a wholesome and delicious breakfast that is perfect for weekend brunch.

Day 25: Veggie Breakfast Wrap with Scrambled Eggs and Hummus

Cooking Time: 10 minutes

Calories: 350-400

Fill a whole grain wrap with scrambled eggs, sliced cucumber, shredded carrots, and a dollop of hummus for a nutritious and portable breakfast option that is packed with flavor and texture.

Day 26: Banana Bread Overnight Oats

Preparation Time: 5 minutes (+overnight)

Calories: 300-350

Mix rolled oats with mashed banana, almond milk, cinnamon, and a sprinkle of walnuts. Let sit overnight in the refrigerator and top with sliced banana for a creamy and satisfying breakfast that taste

Day 27: Spinach and Mushroom Breakfast Quesadilla

Cooking Time: 10 minutes

Calories: 300-350

Sauté spinach and mushrooms until tender. Spread onto a whole grain tortilla, sprinkle with shredded cheese, and fold in half. Cook until golden brown on both sides, and then slice into wedges for a savory and satisfying breakfast.

Day 28: Protein-Packed Breakfast Cookies with Collagen Powder

Cooking Time: 20 minutes

Calories: 150-200 (per cookie)

Bake homemade breakfast cookies using rolled oats, mashed banana, collagen powder, and your choice of nuts or seeds. Enjoy these nutrient-dense cookies for a convenient and on-the-go breakfast option.

Day 29: Egg and Avocado Breakfast Salad with Lemon Vinaigrette

Preparation Time: 10 minutes

Calories: 300-350

Toss mixed greens with sliced avocado, hard-boiled eggs, cherry tomatoes, and a homemade lemon vinaigrette made with olive oil, lemon juice, and Dijon mustard. Serve as a refreshing and nutritious salad to start your day.

Day 30: Coconut Chia Seed Pancakes with Raspberry Compote

Cooking Time: 15 minutes

Calories: 300-350

Make coconut chia seed pancakes and serve with a homemade raspberry compote made by simmering fresh or frozen raspberries with a splash of maple syrup. Top with a dollop of Greek yogurt for a decadent and satisfying breakfast treat.

With these additional breakfast options, you have a full month's worth of delicious and collagen-boosting meals to enjoy. Feel free to mix and match these recipes based on your preferences and dietary needs, and start each day with a nutritious and energizing breakfast that supports your health and well-being.

30 DAYS OF HEALTHY LUNCH OPTIONS:

Day 1: Grilled Chicken Salad

Cooking Time: 20 minutes

Calories: 350-400

Description: Marinate chicken breasts in lemon juice, olive oil, and herbs, then grill until cooked through. Serve sliced over a bed of mixed greens with cherry tomatoes, cucumber, red onion, and a balsamic vinaigrette for a refreshing and protein-packed salad.

Day 2: Quinoa and Black Bean Buddha Bowl

Cooking Time: 25 minutes

Calories: 400-450

Description: Cook quinoa according to package instructions and serve with black beans, roasted sweet potatoes, sautéed kale, avocado slices, and a drizzle of tahini dressing. This nutrient-dense Buddha bowl is packed with plant-based protein and fiber to keep you feeling satisfied all afternoon.

Day 3: Turkey and Avocado Wrap

Preparation Time: 10 minutes

Calories: 300-350

Description: Spread a whole grain tortilla with mashed avocado, layer with sliced turkey breast, spinach leaves, shredded carrots, and cucumber sticks. Roll up tightly and slice in half for a quick and portable lunch option that is perfect for on the go.

Day 4: Lentil Soup with Whole Grain Bread

Cooking Time: 30 minutes

Calories: 300-350

Description: Simmer lentils with carrots, celery, onions, garlic, and vegetable broth until tender. Season with herbs and spices, and then serve with a slice of whole grain bread for a comforting and nutritious soup that is high in fiber and protein.

Day 5: Tuna Salad Sandwich

Preparation Time: 10 minutes

Calories: 350-400

Description: Mix canned tuna with Greek yogurt, diced celery, red onion, and dill. Spread onto whole grain bread and top with lettuce leaves and tomato slices for a classic and protein-packed sandwich that is perfect for lunchtime.

Day 6: Veggie Stir-Fry with Tofu

Cooking Time: 15 minutes

Calories: 300-350

Description: Sauté tofu cubes with broccoli florets, bell peppers, snap peas, and mushrooms in a flavorful stir-fry sauce made with soy sauce, ginger, and garlic. Serve over brown rice or quinoa for a satisfying and veggie-packed lunch option.

Day 7: Chickpea and Spinach Salad with Lemon Vinaigrette

Preparation Time: 15 minutes

Calories: 350-400

Description: Combine chickpeas, baby spinach, cherry tomatoes, cucumber slices, and crumbled feta cheese in a large bowl. Drizzle with a homemade lemon vinaigrette made with olive oil, lemon juice, Dijon mustard, and honey for a refreshing and protein-rich salad.

Day 8: Mediterranean Quinoa Salad

Cooking Time: 20 minutes

Calories: 350-400

Description: Toss cooked quinoa with diced cucumber, cherry tomatoes, Kalamata olives, red onion, and crumbled feta cheese. Dress with a lemon-herb vinaigrette and serve chilled for a light and flavorful lunch option inspired by Mediterranean cuisine.

Day 9: Grilled Salmon with Roasted Vegetables

Cooking Time: 25 minutes

Calories: 400-450

Description: Marinate salmon fillets in a mixture of olive oil, lemon zest, garlic, and herbs, then grill until cooked through. Serve with roasted vegetables such as asparagus, bell peppers, and zucchini for a protein-packed and nutrient-rich lunch.

Day 10: Chicken Caesar Salad

Preparation Time: 15 minutes

Calories: 350-400

Description: Toss chopped romaine lettuce with grilled chicken breast slices, Parmesan cheese, and whole grain croutons. Dress with a homemade Caesar dressing made with Greek yogurt, lemon juice, garlic, and anchovies for a satisfying and flavorful salad.

Day 11: Black Bean and Sweet Potato Quesadilla

Cooking Time: 20 minutes

Calories: 350-400

Description: Mash cooked sweet potatoes and spread onto a whole grain tortilla. Top with black beans, shredded cheese, and sliced jalapeños, then fold in half and cook until crispy and golden brown for a hearty and vegetarian-friendly quesadilla.

Day 12: Capers Panini with Tomato Soup

Cooking Time: 15 minutes

Calories: 400-450

Description: Layer sliced mozzarella cheese, tomato slices, and fresh basil leaves between whole grain bread slices. Grill until the cheese is melted and the bread is toasted, and then serve with a side of homemade tomato soup for a comforting and classic lunchtime combination.

Day 13: Shrimp and Avocado Salad

Preparation Time: 15 minutes

Calories: 300-350

Description: Toss cooked shrimp with mixed greens, diced avocado, cherry tomatoes, and cucumber slices. Dress with a lime-cilantro vinaigrette and sprinkle with toasted pepitas for a light and refreshing salad that is rich in protein and healthy fats.

Day 14: Vegetable and Lentil Curry with Brown Rice

Cooking Time: 30 minutes

Calories: 350-400

Description: Simmer lentils with coconut milk, diced tomatoes, and curry spices until tender. Add chopped vegetables such as carrots, bell peppers, and cauliflower, and cook until softened. Serve over brown rice for a hearty and flavorful vegetarian curry.

Day 15: Greek Chicken Pita Pocket

Preparation Time: 15 minutes

Calories: 350-400

Description: Stuff whole-wheat pita pockets with grilled chicken strips, cucumber slices, cherry tomatoes, red onion, and tzatziki sauce. Serve with a side of Greek salad for a fresh and satisfying lunch option inspired by Mediterranean flavors.

Day 16: Eggplant Parmesan with Whole Wheat Pasta

Cooking Time: 30 minutes

Calories: 400-450

Description: Bread and bake eggplant slices until golden brown, then layer with marinara sauce, mozzarella cheese, and Parmesan cheese. Serve over whole-wheat pasta for a vegetarian twist on the classic Italian dish that is hearty and satisfying.

Day 17: Asian Beef and Broccoli Stir-Fry

Cooking Time: 20 minutes

Calories: 400-450

Description: Sauté thinly sliced beef with broccoli florets, bell peppers, and snap peas in a flavorful stir-fry sauce made with soy sauce, ginger, garlic, and sesame oil. Serve over brown rice for a quick and delicious Asian-inspired lunch option.

Day 18: Quinoa Stuffed Bell Peppers

Cooking Time: 30 minutes

Calories: 350-400

Description: Cut bell peppers in half and remove seeds, then stuff with a mixture of cooked quinoa, black beans, corn, diced tomatoes, and spices. Bake until the peppers are tender and the filling is heated through for a colorful and nutritious vegetarian meal.

Day 19: Spinach and Mushroom Quesadilla

Cooking Time: 15 minutes

Calories: 300-350

Description: Sauté spinach and sliced mushrooms with garlic until wilted. Spread the mixture onto a whole grain tortilla, sprinkle with shredded cheese, and fold in half. Cook on a skillet until the tortilla is crispy and the cheese is melted for a quick and savory lunch option.

Day 20: Turkey and Veggie Wrap

Preparation Time: 10 minutes

Calories: 350-400

Description: Spread hummus onto a whole-wheat wrap, layer with sliced turkey breast, shredded lettuce, grated carrots, cucumber slices, and avocado. Roll up tightly and slice in half for a nutritious and portable lunch option that is packed with protein and veggies.

Day 21: Chicken Fajita Bowl

Cooking Time: 25 minutes

Calories: 400-450

Description: Sauté sliced chicken breast with bell peppers, onions, and fajita seasoning until cooked through. Serve over brown rice or quinoa, and top with salsa, guacamole, and Greek yogurt for a flavorful and satisfying lunch bowl inspired by Tex-Mex cuisine.

Day 22: Mediterranean Chickpea Salad

Preparation Time: 15 minutes

Calories: 350-400

Description: Combine chickpeas, diced cucumber, cherry tomatoes, red onion, Kalamata olives, and crumbled feta cheese in a large bowl. Dress with a lemon-herb vinaigrette and sprinkle with fresh parsley for a refreshing and protein-rich salad that is perfect for a light lunch.

Day 23: Pesto Pasta with Cherry Tomatoes and Mozzarella

Cooking Time: 20 minutes

Calories: 400-450

Description: Cook whole-wheat pasta according to package instructions, then toss with homemade pesto sauce, halved cherry tomatoes, fresh mozzarella balls, and toasted pine nuts. Serve warm or chilled for a delicious and flavorful pasta salad that is perfect for lunch.

Day 24: Salmon and Avocado Sushi Rolls

Cooking Time: 30 minutes

Calories: 350-400

Description: Cook sushi rice according to package instructions and season with rice vinegar and sugar. Spread onto nori sheets, and then layer with sliced avocado and cooked salmon. Roll tightly and slice into sushi rolls for a homemade and nutritious lunch option that is perfect for sushi lovers.

Day 25: Thai Peanut Chicken Wrap

Preparation Time: 15 minutes

Calories: 350-400

Description: Spread peanut sauce onto a whole-wheat wrap, layer with sliced grilled chicken breast, shredded cabbage, shredded carrots, chopped cilantro, and sliced red bell pepper. Roll up tightly and slice in half for a flavorful and satisfying lunch wrap with a Thai-inspired twist.

Day 26: Quinoa and Kale Salad with Lemon Tahini Dressing

Preparation Time: 20 minutes

Calories: 350-400

Description: Toss cooked quinoa with chopped kale, shredded Brussels sprouts, dried cranberries, toasted almonds, and crumbled feta cheese in a large bowl. Dress with a creamy lemon tahini dressing made with tahini, lemon juice, garlic, and olive oil for a nutritious and flavorful salad option.

Day 27: Veggie Burger with Sweet Potato Fries

Cooking Time: 25 minutes

Calories: 400-450

Description: Grill or bake veggie burgers until heated through, then serve on whole grain buns with lettuce, tomato, red onion, and avocado slices. Serve with baked sweet potato fries for a satisfying and plant-based lunch option that is perfect for burger lovers.

Day 28: Chicken and Vegetable Stir-Fry with Rice Noodles

Cooking Time: 20 minutes

Calories: 400-450

Description: Stir-fry sliced chicken breast with mixed vegetables such as bell peppers, snap peas, carrots, and broccoli in a flavorful sauce made with soy sauce, ginger, garlic, and sesame oil. Serve over cooked rice noodles for a quick and delicious Asian-inspired lunch option.

Day 29: Mediterranean Hummus Wrap

Preparation Time: 10 minutes

Calories: 300-350

Description: Spread hummus onto a whole-wheat wrap, layer with diced cucumber, cherry tomatoes, red onion, Kalamata olives, and crumbled feta cheese. Roll up tightly and slice in half for a flavorful and satisfying wrap that is perfect for a light lunch.

Day 30: Beef and Broccoli Noodle Bowl

Cooking Time: 25 minutes

Calories: 400-450

Description: Sauté thinly sliced beef with broccoli florets and sliced carrots in a savory sauce made with soy sauce, ginger, and garlic.

30 DAYS NUTRITIOUS DINNER OPTIONS

Day 1: Baked Lemon Herb Salmon with Roasted Vegetables

Cooking Time: 25 minutes

Calories: 400-450

Description: Marinate salmon fillets in a mixture of lemon juice, olive oil, garlic, and herbs, then bake until tender and flaky. Serve with a side of roasted vegetables such as carrots, broccoli, and cauliflower for a flavorful and nutritious dinner.

Day 2: Vegetarian Chickpea Curry with Basmati Rice

Cooking Time: 30 minutes

Calories: 350-400

Description: Sauté onions, garlic, and ginger until fragrant, then add chickpeas, diced tomatoes, coconut milk, and curry spices. Simmer until the flavors meld together, and then serve over cooked basmati rice for a comforting and satisfying vegetarian curry.

Day 3: Grilled Chicken Breast with Quinoa and Steamed Broccoli

Cooking Time: 25 minutes

Calories: 400-450

Description: Marinate chicken breasts in a mixture of olive oil, lemon juice, garlic, and herbs, then grill until cooked through. Serve with a side of cooked quinoa and steamed broccoli for a protein-packed and nutritious dinner option.

Day 4: Beef Stir-Fry with Mixed Vegetables and Brown Rice

Cooking Time: 20 minutes

Calories: 400-450

Description: Stir-fry thinly sliced beef with mixed vegetables such as bell peppers, snap peas, carrots, and broccoli in a flavorful sauce made with soy sauce, ginger, garlic, and sesame oil. Serve over cooked brown rice for a quick and delicious dinner.

Day 5: Caprese Stuffed Portobello Mushrooms

Cooking Time: 30 minutes

Calories: 350-400

Description: Remove the stems from portobello mushrooms and fill the caps with sliced tomatoes, fresh mozzarella cheese, and basil leaves. Drizzle with balsamic glaze and bake until the mushrooms are tender and the cheese is melted for a vegetarian-friendly dinner option.

Day 6: Spaghetti Squash with Turkey Bolognese Sauce

Cooking Time: 45 minutes

Calories: 350-400

Description: Roast spaghetti squash until tender, and then shred the flesh with a fork to create "noodles". Serve with a homemade turkey Bolognese sauce made with lean ground turkey, diced tomatoes, garlic, and herbs for a lighter twist on a classic pasta dish.

Day 7: Veggie-packed Minestrone Soup with Garlic Bread

Cooking Time: 40 minutes

Calories: 300-350

Description: Simmer diced vegetables such as carrots, celery, zucchini, and green beans with canned tomatoes, vegetable broth, and pasta until tender. Serve with a side of garlic bread for a hearty and comforting soup that is perfect for a cozy dinner.

Day 8: Honey Garlic Glazed Shrimp with Stir-Fried Vegetables

Cooking Time: 20 minutes

Calories: 350-400

Description: Sauté shrimp with minced garlic until pink and opaque, then toss with a homemade honey garlic glaze made with honey, soy sauce, and ginger. Serve with a side of stir-fried vegetables such as bell peppers, snap peas, and carrots for a quick and flavorful dinner.

Day 9: Mediterranean Baked Chicken with Greek Salad

Cooking Time: 30 minutes

Calories: 400-450

Description: Marinate chicken breasts in a mixture of olive oil, lemon juice, garlic, and herbs, and then bake until cooked through. Serve with a side of Greek salad made with cucumbers, tomatoes, red onion, Kalamata olives, and feta cheese for a refreshing and flavorful dinner.

Day 10: Quinoa Stuffed Bell Peppers with Side Salad

Cooking Time: 35 minutes

Calories: 350-400

Description: Cut bell peppers in half and remove seeds, then stuff with a mixture of cooked quinoa, black beans, corn, diced tomatoes, and spices. Bake until the peppers are tender and the filling is heated through, and then serve with a side salad for a nutritious and satisfying vegetarian meal.

Day 11: Teriyaki Tofu Stir-Fry with Brown Rice

Cooking Time: 25 minutes

Calories: 350-400

Description: Stir-fry cubed tofu with mixed vegetables such as broccoli, bell peppers, snap peas, and carrots in a homemade teriyaki sauce made with soy sauce, ginger, garlic, and honey. Serve over cooked brown rice for a delicious and plant-based dinner option.

Day 12: Lemon Herb Grilled Chicken with Roasted Asparagus

Cooking Time: 25 minutes

Calories: 400-450

Description: Marinate chicken breasts in a mixture of lemon juice, olive oil, garlic, and herbs, then grill until cooked through. Serve with a side of roasted asparagus spears drizzled with olive oil and sprinkled with lemon zest for a light and flavorful dinner.

Day 13: Lentil Shepherd's Pie with Mashed Sweet Potatoes

Cooking Time: 40 minutes

Calories: 350-400

Description: Sauté onions, carrots, and celery until softened, then add cooked lentils, diced tomatoes, and herbs. Simmer until heated through, then transfer to a baking dish and top with mashed sweet potatoes. Bake until golden and bubbly for a hearty and comforting vegetarian shepherd's pie.

Day 14: Shrimp and Avocado Salad with Creamy Cilantro Dressing

Cooking Time: 20 minutes

Calories: 350-400

Description: Sauté shrimp with minced garlic until pink and opaque, then serve over a bed of mixed greens with sliced avocado, cherry tomatoes, and sliced red onion. Drizzle with a creamy cilantro dressing made with Greek yogurt, limejuice, cilantro, and garlic for a refreshing and protein-packed salad that is perfect for a light dinner.

Day 15: Veggie-loaded Turkey Chili with Cornbread Muffins

Cooking Time: 45 minutes

Calories: 350-400

Description: Cook ground turkey with onions, bell peppers, and garlic until brown, and then add diced tomatoes, kidney beans, corn, and spices. Simmer until the flavors meld together, and then serve with a side of cornbread muffins for a comforting and hearty dinner option.

Day 16: Balsamic Glazed Pork Chops with Roasted Brussels Sprouts

Cooking Time: 30 minutes

Calories: 400-450

Description: Marinate pork chops in a mixture of balsamic vinegar, honey, garlic, and herbs, then grill or bake until cooked through. Serve with a side of roasted Brussels sprouts tossed with olive oil, balsamic vinegar, and garlic for a flavorful and nutritious dinner.

Day 17: Cauliflower Crust Pizza with Salad

Cooking Time: 30 minutes

Calories: 350-400

Description: Top a cauliflower crust with marinara sauce, shredded mozzarella cheese, and your favorite pizza toppings such as bell peppers, onions, and mushrooms. Bake until the crust is crispy and the cheese is melted, and then serve with a side salad for a lighter twist on pizza night.

Day 18: Thai Red Curry with Tofu and Jasmine Rice

Cooking Time: 30 minutes

Calories: 400-450

Description: Sauté cubed tofu with mixed vegetables such as bell peppers, snap peas, and carrots in a flavorful Thai red curry sauce made with coconut milk, red curry paste, and ginger. Serve over cooked jasmine rice for a delicious and aromatic dinner option.

Day 19: Mediterranean Stuffed Zucchini Boats

Cooking Time: 35 minutes

Calories: 350-400

Description: Cut zucchini in half lengthwise and scoop out the seeds to create "boats". Fill with a mixture of cooked quinoa, chickpeas, cherry tomatoes, Kalamata olives, and feta cheese. Bake until the zucchini is tender and the filling is heated through for a flavorful and nutritious vegetarian meal.

Day 20: Lemon Garlic Shrimp Pasta with Spinach

Cooking Time: 20 minutes

Calories: 400-450

Description: Sauté shrimp with minced garlic until pink and opaque, then toss with cooked pasta, baby spinach, lemon zest, and Parmesan cheese. Serve with a side of garlic bread for a quick and delicious dinner option that is bursting with flavor.

Day 21: Honey Mustard Glazed Salmon with Quinoa Pilaf

Cooking Time: 25 minutes

Calories: 400-450

Description: Marinate salmon fillets in a mixture of honey, Dijon mustard, and lemon juice, then bake until cooked through. Serve with a side of quinoa pilaf made with diced vegetables and herbs for a flavorful and protein-packed dinner.

Day 22: Vegetable Pad Thai with Tofu

Cooking Time: 25 minutes

Calories: 350-400

Description: Stir-fry cubed tofu with mixed vegetables such as bean sprouts, bell peppers, and carrots in a tangy Pad Thai sauce made with tamarind paste, soy sauce, and lime juice. Serve over cooked rice noodles and garnish with chopped peanuts and cilantro for a delicious and satisfying dinner.

Day 23: Chicken and Vegetable Skewers with Herbed Couscous

Cooking Time: 30 minutes

Calories: 400-450

Description: Thread cubed chicken breast and mixed vegetables such as bell peppers, zucchini, and onions onto skewers, then grill or bake until cooked through. Serve with a side of herbed couscous made with fresh herbs and lemon zest for a flavorful and protein-packed dinner option.

Day 24: Butternut Squash and Black Bean Enchiladas

Cooking Time: 40 minutes

Calories: 350-400

Description: Fill corn tortillas with a mixture of roasted butternut squash, black beans, diced tomatoes, and spices. Roll up and place in a baking dish, then top with enchilada sauce and cheese. Bake until bubbly and golden for a delicious and satisfying vegetarian dinner.

Day 25: Ratatouille with Garlic Bread

Cooking Time: 35 minutes

Calories: 350-400

Description: Sauté diced eggplant, zucchini, bell peppers, and tomatoes with garlic and herbs until tender, then serve with a side of garlic bread for a flavorful and comforting French-inspired dinner option.

Day 26: Greek Lemon Chicken with Orzo and Roasted Vegetables

Cooking Time: 40 minutes

Calories: 400-450

Description: Marinate chicken thighs in a mixture of lemon juice, olive oil, garlic, and oregano, and then bake until cooked through. Serve with a side of cooked orzo and roasted vegetables such as bell peppers, onions, and cherry tomatoes for a delicious and Mediterranean-inspired dinner.

Day 27: Lentil and Vegetable Curry with Naan Bread

Cooking Time: 35 minutes

Calories: 350-400

Description: Simmer lentils with mixed vegetables such as carrots, potatoes, and spinach in a flavorful curry sauce made with coconut milk and spices. Serve with a side of naan bread for a comforting and satisfying vegetarian dinner.

Day 28: BBQ Jackfruit Sandwiches with Coleslaw

Cooking Time: 30 minutes

Calories: 350-400

Description: Sauté shredded jackfruit with barbecue sauce until heated through, and then serve on whole grain buns with a side of homemade coleslaw made with shredded cabbage, carrots, and Greek yogurt dressing for a delicious and plant-based dinner option.

Day 29: Stuffed Acorn Squash with Wild Rice Pilaf

Cooking Time: 45 minutes

Calories: 350-400

Description: Cut acorn squash in half and remove seeds, then fill with a mixture of cooked wild rice, dried cranberries, chopped pecans, and herbs.

Day 30: Grilled Chicken with Roasted Sweet Potatoes and Steamed Broccoli

Cooking Time: 40 minutes

Calories: 350-400 per serving

Description: Season chicken breasts with your favorite herbs and grill until cooked through. Serve with roasted sweet potato wedges seasoned with paprika and garlic powder, and steamed broccoli on the side.

30 DAYS HEARTY SNACK OPTIONS
Day 1: Greek Yogurt Parfait with Berries and Granola

Calories: Approximately 250-300 per serving

Preparation Time: 5 minutes

Description: Layer Greek yogurt with fresh berries and granola for a creamy, fruity, and crunchy snack that is packed with protein and fiber.

Day 2: Apple Slices with Almond Butter

Calories: Approximately 150-200 per serving

Preparation Time: 2 minutes

Description: Spread almond butter on apple slices for a satisfying and nutritious snack that combines the sweetness of fruit with the creaminess of nut butter.

Day 3: Veggie Sticks with Hummus

Calories: Approximately 100-150 per serving

Preparation Time: 5 minutes

Description: Dip carrot, cucumber, and bell pepper sticks into creamy hummus for a crunchy, refreshing, and protein-rich snack that is perfect for dipping.

Day 4: Trail Mix with Nuts, Seeds, and Dried Fruit

Calories: Approximately 200-250 per serving

Preparation Time: 5 minutes

Description: Mix a variety of nuts, seeds, and dried fruit for a portable and energy-boosting snack that provides a satisfying mix of sweet and savory flavors.

Day 5: Cottage Cheese with Pineapple Chunks

Calories: Approximately 150-200 per serving

Preparation Time: 2 minutes

Description: Top cottage cheese with pineapple chunks for a creamy and tropical snack that is rich in protein, calcium, and vitamin C.

Day 6: Rice Cakes with Avocado and Tomato Slices

Calories: Approximately 150-200 per serving

Preparation Time: 5 minutes

Description: Spread mashed avocado on rice cakes and top with sliced tomatoes for a crunchy and satisfying snack that is packed with healthy fats and vitamins.

Day 7: Edamame with Sea Salt

Calories: Approximately 100-150 per serving

Preparation Time: 10 minutes

Description: Enjoy steamed edamame sprinkled with sea salt for a tasty and protein-packed snack that is perfect for satisfying mid-afternoon cravings.

Day 8: Greek Yogurt with Honey and Walnuts

Calories: Approximately 200-250 per serving

Preparation Time: 2 minutes

Description: Drizzle Greek yogurt with honey and sprinkle with chopped walnuts for a creamy, sweet, and crunchy snack that is rich in protein and healthy fats.

Day 9: Whole Grain Crackers with Cheese Slices

Calories: Approximately 200-250 per serving

Preparation Time: 2 minutes

Description: Pair whole grain crackers with cheese slices for a satisfying and balanced snack that provides a mix of carbohydrates, protein, and calcium.

Day 10: Popcorn with Nutritional Yeast

Calories: Approximately 100-150 per serving

Preparation Time: 5 minutes

Description: Sprinkle air-popped popcorn with nutritional yeast for a cheesy and flavorful snack that is low in calories and high in fiber.

Day 11: Banana with Peanut Butter and Dark Chocolate Chips

Calories: Approximately 200-250 per serving

Preparation Time: 2 minutes

Description: Spread peanut butter on banana slices and top with dark chocolate chips for a sweet and indulgent snack that is satisfying and nutritious.

Day 12: Hard-Boiled Eggs with Everything Bagel Seasoning

Calories: Approximately 150-200 per serving

Preparation Time: 15 minutes

Description: Sprinkle hard-boiled eggs with everything bagel seasoning for a flavorful and protein-rich snack that is easy to make and enjoy on the go.

Day 13: Greek Yogurt Dip with Veggie Chips

Calories: Approximately 150-200 per serving

Preparation Time: 5 minutes

Description: Serve Greek yogurt dip with homemade or store-bought veggie chips for a crunchy and satisfying snack that is perfect for dipping.

Day 14: Rice Cakes with Hummus and Sliced Cucumber

Calories: Approximately 150-200 per serving

Preparation Time: 5 minutes

Description: Spread hummus on rice cakes and top with sliced cucumber for a light and refreshing snack that is crunchy, creamy, and full of flavor.

Day 15: Mixed Berries with Cottage Cheese

Calories: Approximately 150-200 per serving

Preparation Time: 2 minutes

Description: Enjoy a bowl of mixed berries with cottage cheese for a creamy and antioxidant-rich snack that is perfect for satisfying sweet cravings.

Day 16: Almonds with Dried Apricots

Calories: Approximately 150-200 per serving

Preparation Time: 2 minutes

Description: Pair almonds with dried apricots for a sweet and crunchy snack that is rich in protein, fiber, and essential nutrients.

Day 17: Celery Sticks with Peanut Butter and Raisins

Calories: Approximately 150-200 per serving

Preparation Time: 5 minutes

Description: Fill celery sticks with peanut butter and top with raisins for a crunchy, creamy, and naturally sweet snack that is satisfying and nutritious.

Day 18: Whole Grain Toast with Avocado and Sliced Tomato

Calories: Approximately 200-250 per serving

Preparation Time: 5 minutes

Description: Top whole grain toast with mashed avocado and sliced tomato for a hearty and satisfying snack that is packed with fiber, healthy fats, and vitamins.

Day 19: Yogurt Bark with Mixed Nuts and Dried Fruit

Calories: Approximately 200-250 per serving

Preparation Time: 15 minutes (plus freezing time)

Description: Spread Greek yogurt onto a baking sheet, then sprinkle with mixed nuts and dried fruit before freezing for a refreshing and nutritious snack that is perfect for hot days.

Day 20: Cottage Cheese with Sliced Peaches

Calories: Approximately 150-200 per serving

Preparation Time: 2 minutes

Description: Pair cottage cheese with sliced peaches for a creamy, fruity, and protein-packed snack that is perfect for a quick and easy refreshment.

Day 21: Hummus with Whole Grain Pita Bread

Calories: Approximately 150-200 per serving

Preparation Time: 5 minutes

Description: Dip whole grain pita bread into creamy hummus for a satisfying and fiber-rich snack that is perfect for satisfying hunger between meals.

Day 22: Greek Yogurt with Chia Seeds and Honey

Calories: Approximately 200-250 per serving

Preparation Time: 2 minutes

Description: Stir chia seeds and honey into Greek yogurt for a creamy and nutritious snack that is rich in protein, fiber, and omega-3 fatty acids.

Day 23: Almond Butter with Banana Slices on Rice Cakes

Calories: Approximately 200-250 per serving

Preparation Time: 2 minutes

Description: Spread almond butter on rice cakes and top with banana slices for a crunchy, creamy, and naturally sweet snack that is perfect for satisfying cravings.

Day 24: Veggie Sticks with Greek Yogurt Ranch Dip

Calories: Approximately 100-150 per serving

Preparation Time: 5 minutes

Description: Serve crunchy veggie sticks with creamy Greek yogurt ranch dip for a refreshing and nutritious snack that is perfect for dipping.

Day 25: Popcorn with Cinnamon and Maple Syrup

Calories: Approximately 100-150 per serving

Preparation Time: 5 minutes

Description: Drizzle air-popped popcorn with cinnamon and maple syrup for a sweet and satisfying snack that is perfect for satisfying sweet cravings without added sugar.

Day 26: Cheese and Crackers with Grapes

Calories: Approximately 200-250 per serving

Preparation Time: 2 minutes

Description: Pair cheese and whole grain crackers with grapes for a balanced and satisfying snack that provides a mix of protein, carbohydrates, and vitamins.

Day 27: Apple Slices with Cottage Cheese and Cinnamon

Calories: Approximately 150-200 per serving

Preparation Time: 2 minutes

Description: Top apple slices with cottage cheese and sprinkle with cinnamon for a creamy, sweet, and satisfying snack that is perfect for satisfying hunger between meals.

Day 28: Greek Yogurt with Pumpkin Seeds and Honey

Calories: Approximately 200-250 per serving

Preparation Time: 2 minutes

Description: Sprinkle pumpkin seeds and drizzle honey over Greek yogurt for a creamy, crunchy, and naturally sweet snack that is rich in protein, fiber, and essential nutrients.

Day 29: Carrot Sticks with Hummus and Sunflower Seeds

Calories: Approximately 100-150 per serving

Preparation Time: 5 minutes

Description: Dip carrot sticks into hummus and sprinkle with sunflower seeds for a crunchy, creamy, and protein-rich snack that is perfect for satisfying hunger between meals.

Day 30: Rice Cakes with Cottage Cheese and Sliced Strawberries

Calories: Approximately 150-200 per serving

Preparation Time: 2 minutes

Description: Spread cottage cheese on rice cakes and top with sliced strawberries for a refreshing, creamy, and protein-packed snack that is perfect for satisfying sweet cravings.

These snack options provide a variety of flavors, textures, and nutrients to keep you satisfied and energized throughout the day. Adjust portion sizes and ingredients based on personal preferences and dietary needs.

30 DAYS OF YUMMY DESSERT AND TREAT OPTIONS

Day 1: Dark Chocolate Covered Strawberries

Calories: 50-100 per strawberry

Preparation Time: 15 minutes

Description: Dip fresh strawberries in melted dark chocolate and let them set in the refrigerator until the chocolate hardens for a sweet and indulgent treat.

Day 2: Frozen Banana Pops

Calories: 100-150 per banana

Preparation Time: 20 minutes

Description: Insert Popsicle sticks into peeled bananas, dip them in melted chocolate, sprinkle with chopped nuts or coconut flakes, and freeze until firm for a delicious and satisfying frozen treat.

Day 3: Greek Yogurt Bark with Berries and Almonds

Calories: 150-200 per serving

Preparation Time: 10 minutes + freezing time

Description: Spread Greek yogurt onto a baking sheet, top with fresh berries and chopped almonds, and freeze until firm. Break into pieces and enjoy as a creamy and nutritious dessert.

Day 4: Baked Apples with Cinnamon and Walnuts

Calories: 100-150 per apple

Preparation Time: 30 minutes

Description: Core apples, sprinkle with cinnamon and chopped walnuts, and bake until tender for a warm and comforting dessert that is naturally sweet and delicious.

Day 5: Chocolate Avocado Mousse

Calories: 150-200 per serving

Preparation Time: 10 minutes

Description: Blend ripe avocados with cocoa powder, maple syrup, and vanilla extract until smooth and creamy. Chill in the refrigerator before serving for a rich and decadent dessert.

Day 6: Chia Seed Pudding with Mixed Berries

Calories: 150-200 per serving

Preparation Time: 5 minutes + chilling time

Description: Mix chia seeds with almond milk, vanilla extract, and a sweetener of choice, then let it sit in the refrigerator until thickened. Serve with fresh berries for a creamy and nutritious pudding.

Day 7: Frozen Yogurt Bark with Mango and Coconut

Calories: 150-200 per serving

Preparation Time: 10 minutes + freezing time

Description: Spread Greek yogurt onto a baking sheet, top with diced mango and shredded coconut, and freeze until firm. Break into pieces and enjoy as a refreshing and tropical dessert.

Day 8: Grilled Peaches with Honey and Greek Yogurt

Calories: 100-150 per serving

Preparation Time: 15 minutes

Description: Halve peaches and grill until tender, then drizzle with honey and serve with a dollop of Greek yogurt for a simple yet elegant dessert that is bursting with flavor.

Day 9: Coconut Chia Popsicles

Calories: 100-150 per Popsicle

Preparation Time: 10 minutes + freezing time

Description: Blend coconut milk with chia seeds, maple syrup, and vanilla extract, then pour into Popsicle molds and freeze until solid for a creamy and refreshing frozen treat.

Day 10: Almond Butter Stuffed Dates

Calories: 50-100 per date

Preparation Time: 5 minutes

Description: Pit Medjool dates and fill them with almond butter for a sweet and satisfying snack that is perfect for satisfying sweet cravings.

Day 11: Berry Coconut Parfait

Calories: 150-200 per serving

Preparation Time: 5 minutes

Description: Layer mixed berries with coconut yogurt and granola for a colorful and refreshing parfait that is perfect for a light and satisfying dessert.

Day 12: Frozen Chocolate Banana Bites

Calories: 100-150 per serving

Preparation Time: 15 minutes + freezing time

Description: Slice bananas, dip them in melted chocolate, and freeze until firm for a sweet and creamy frozen treat that is perfect for satisfying chocolate cravings.

Day 13: Lemon Poppy Seed Muffins

Calories: 150-200 per muffin

Preparation Time: 30 minutes

Description: Bake lemon poppy seed muffins until golden and fragrant for a zesty and satisfying treat that is perfect for breakfast or dessert.

Day 14: Mixed Berry Crisp

Calories: 200-250 per serving

Preparation Time: 45 minutes

Description: Toss mixed berries with a squeeze of lemon juice and a sprinkle of sugar, then top with a mixture of oats, almond flour, coconut oil, and maple syrup and bake until bubbly and golden for a sweet and comforting dessert.

Day 15: Chocolate Covered Frozen Bananas

Calories: 100-150 per banana

Preparation Time: 20 minutes + freezing time

Description: Insert Popsicle sticks into peeled bananas, dip them in melted chocolate, sprinkle with chopped nuts or shredded coconut, and freeze until firm for a creamy and indulgent frozen treat.

Day 16: Raspberry Coconut Chia Pudding

Calories: 150-200 per serving

Preparation Time: 5 minutes + chilling time

Description: Mix chia seeds with coconut milk, raspberries, and a sweetener of choice, then let it sit in the refrigerator until thickened. Serve with a sprinkle of shredded coconut for a creamy and nutritious dessert.

Day 17: Banana Bread Bites

Calories: 100-150 per serving

Preparation Time: 30 minutes

Description: Bake mini banana bread muffins until golden and fragrant for a delicious and portable snack or dessert.

Day 18: Mango Coconut Sorbet

Calories: 100-150 per serving

Preparation Time: 10 minutes + freezing time

Description: Blend frozen mango chunks with coconut milk and a squeeze of lime juice until smooth, then freeze until firm for a refreshing and tropical sorbet that is bursting with flavor.

Day 19: Peanut Butter Chocolate Chip Energy Bites

Calories: 100-150 per serving

Preparation Time: 15 minutes

Description: Mix rolled oats with peanut butter, honey, and chocolate chips, then roll into bite-sized balls and chill until firm for a satisfying and energy-boosting snack or dessert.

Day 20: Lemon Blueberry Scones

Calories: 150-200 per scone

Preparation Time: 30 minutes

Description: Bake lemon blueberry scones until golden and fragrant for a light and flaky treat that is perfect for breakfast or dessert.

Day 21: Coconut Mango Rice Pudding

Calories: 150-200 per serving

Preparation Time: 45 minutes

Description: Cook rice with coconut milk, diced mango, and a sweetener of choice until creamy and thickened for a tropical twist on classic rice pudding.

Day 22: Chocolate Almond Butter Cups

Calories: 100-150 per cup

Day 23: Fruit Salad with Honey Lime Dressing

Description: Melt dark chocolate and pour into mini muffin liners, then top with a dollop of almond butter and another layer of melted chocolate for a rich and indulgent treat that is perfect for satisfying chocolate cravings.

Day 23: Fruit Salad with Honey Lime Dressing

Calories: 100-150 per serving

Preparation Time: 10 minutes

Description: Toss together a variety of fresh fruits such as strawberries, kiwi, pineapple, and grapes with a honey lime dressing made with fresh lime juice and honey for a refreshing and naturally sweet dessert.

Day 24: Chocolate Avocado Brownies

Calories: 150-200 per serving

Preparation Time: 40 minutes

Description: Blend ripe avocados with cocoa powder, almond flour, maple syrup, and chocolate chips, and then bake until fudgy and delicious for a healthier twist on traditional brownies.

Day 25: Raspberry Coconut Chia Popsicles

Calories: 100-150 per Popsicle

Preparation Time: 10 minutes + freezing time

Description: Blend coconut milk with raspberries, chia seeds, and a sweetener of choice, then pour into Popsicle molds and freeze until solid for a creamy and refreshing frozen treat.

Day 26: Banana Split with Greek Yogurt

Calories: 150-200 per serving

Preparation Time: 5 minutes

Description: Slice a banana in half lengthwise and top with Greek yogurt, fresh berries, sliced almonds, and a drizzle of honey for a healthier twist on the classic banana split.

Day 27: Peanut Butter Banana Ice Cream

Calories: 150-200 per serving

Preparation Time: 5 minutes

Description: Blend frozen bananas with peanut butter until smooth and creamy, then serve immediately for a delicious and dairy-free ice cream alternative.

Day 28: Strawberry Shortcake Cups

Calories: 150-200 per serving

Preparation Time: 10 minutes

Description: Layer diced strawberries with whipped cream or Greek yogurt and crumbled shortbread cookies in small cups for a light and summery dessert that is perfect for entertaining.

Day 29: Blueberry Lemon Yogurt Popsicles

Calories: 100-150 per Popsicle

Preparation Time: 10 minutes + freezing time

Description: Blend blueberries with Greek yogurt, lemon zest, and honey until smooth, then pour into Popsicle molds and freeze until solid for a refreshing and antioxidant-rich frozen treat.

Day 30: Apple Crisp with Oat Topping

Calories: 150-200 per serving

Preparation Time: 45 minutes

Description: Toss sliced apples with cinnamon and a squeeze of lemon juice, then top with a mixture of oats, almond flour, coconut oil, and maple syrup and bake until bubbly and golden for a comforting and satisfying dessert.

These dessert options provide a variety of flavors and textures to satisfy your sweet cravings while also incorporating nutritious ingredients. Adjust portion sizes and ingredients based on personal preferences and dietary needs. Enjoy experimenting with these recipes!

CHAPTER 6

MAXIMIZING THE BENEFITS OF THE COLLAGEN DIET

Congratulations on starting your collagen diet journey! Collagen, as you have discovered throughout this book, is essential to our general health and wellness. It affects everything from the suppleness of our skin to the strength of our bones and joints. It's time to learn more about how to optimize the benefits of the collagen diet now that you are aware of its fundamentals and have a better understanding of its many facets.

This chapter will cover advanced tactics and methods to maximize the benefits of the collagen diet and make sure you get all of its benefits. Here, we will cover both increasing your body's natural capacity to create and use collagen as well as consuming foods high in the protein.

We will talk about a number of important topics, including how crucial it is to keep up a nutrient-rich, balanced diet in order to promote collagen formation. We will go into detail on the particular vitamins, minerals, and antioxidants that are essential for the synthesis of collagen and how to include them in your diet to support the best possible health for your skin, joints, and bones.

In order to maximize the combined advantages of collagen and other dietary components like protein, healthy fats, and antioxidants, we will also look at the synergistic link between them. You will be more adept at creating meals that encourage collagen synthesis and general wellness if you know how various nutrients interact with collagen in the body.

We will talk about lifestyle factors that can affect collagen production and absorption in addition to dietary issues. We will talk about how your lifestyle decisions can affect the health and integrity of your skin, joints, and connective tissues, from controlling your stress levels and getting enough sleep to staying hydrated and reducing your exposure to environmental pollutants.

We will also explore the function of exercise and physical activity in promoting collagen synthesis and preserving musculoskeletal health. You may protect and improve the flexibility, strength, and resilience of your joints and connective tissues by including specific exercises and movement patterns in your workout regimen.

Finally, we will discuss the possible advantages of taking collagen supplements and how to select collagen products that are high quality and in line with your health objectives. We will offer advice on choosing collagen supplements, such as collagen peptides, bone broth powders, or other items that are produced under strict quality standards and supported by scientific data.

Keep in mind that there is not a one-size-fits-all strategy for optimizing the collagen diet's advantages as you work through this chapter. It is about knowing your own dietary requirements, lifestyle choices, and health goals and adjusting your strategy accordingly. You can achieve robust health and energy from the inside out by adopting a holistic approach to collagen optimization. Together, let us go out on this adventure to fully realize the collagen diet's potential!

Lifestyle Choices that Encourage the Production of Collagen:

Keep Yourself Hydrated: Keeping your skin supple and healthy requires being hydrated. In order to maintain moisturized and plump skin, make sure you consume lots of water throughout the day. In addition to adding to your normal fluid intake, herbal teas and infused water have added antioxidant advantages.

Protect Your Skin from Sun Exposure: Too much sun exposure can hasten the aging process of the skin by breaking down collagen and causing wrinkles, fine lines, and sunspots. Wearing wide spectrum SPF 30 or higher sunscreen, finding shade during the hottest parts of the day, and dressing protectively when you are outside in caps and sunglasses are all good ways to protect your skin.

Have a Well-Balanced Diet: Eating a diet high in nutrients is essential for promoting the formation of collagen and preserving the health of your skin. Your body requires certain vitamins, minerals, and antioxidants to stimulate collagen formation, so make sure your meals include a range of fruits, vegetables, lean meats, healthy fats, and whole grains.

Control Your Stress Levels: Prolonged stress can raise cortisol levels, which over time can cause skin damage and the breakdown of collagen. To encourage relaxation and lower cortisol levels, try stress-reduction methods like yoga, meditation, deep breathing exercises, or spending time in nature.

Get Good Sleep: Sleep is necessary for the renewal and repair of skin. Try to get between seven and nine hours of good sleep every night to give your body time to perform its own healing and renewal processes. To increase the quality of your sleep, establish a nighttime routine, make your sleeping environment as comfortable as possible, and cut back on caffeine and electronics before bed.

Give up Smoking: Smoking causes the skin to age prematurely by hastening the breakdown of collagen. Giving up smoking can enhance general wellbeing, lessen the look of wrinkles, and improve skin health. If you require aid in stopping, seek support from medical specialists or groups designed to help people stop smoking.

Exercise on a Regular Basis: Exercise encourages blood flow, which supports collagen formation and general skin health by supplying nutrients and oxygen to the skin. To maintain maximum musculoskeletal health and skin vibrancy, blend strength training, flexibility training, and cardiovascular activity in your fitness regimen.

Develop Good Skincare Routines: To keep your skin hydrated and healthy, create a skincare regimen that includes gentle washing, moisturizing, and sun protection. To boost collagen formation and retain skin elasticity, look for skincare products that contain components like vitamin C, retinoid, peptides, and hyaluronic acid.

You can encourage the creation of collagen, preserve the health of your skin, and advance general well-being by adopting these lifestyle practices into your everyday routine. For long-term advantages, try incorporating these practices into your daily routine because consistency is essential.

Combining Other Nutrients with Collagen to Achieve Optimal Health:

Collagen is an essential protein that gives the skin, joints, bones, and muscles in the body structural support. While taking collagen supplements can have many positive effects on health, combining collagen with additional nutrients can increase its potency and improve general health and wellbeing. For optimum health, you should think about combining the following essential nutrients with collagen:

Vitamin C: Due to its critical function in the creation of collagen molecules, vitamin C is necessary for the synthesis of collagen. In addition to collagen supplements, eating foods high in vitamin C, such as citrus fruits, strawberries, kiwis, and bell peppers, can increase the formation of collagen and improve joint health, wound healing, and skin health.

Good Fats: Flaxseeds, chia seeds, walnuts, and fatty fish are good sources of omega-3 fatty acids, which have anti-inflammatory qualities that work in tandem with collagen to support and lessen inflammation and promote joint health. Including good fats in your diet in addition to collagen, helps improve cardiovascular, mental, and skin suppleness.

Antioxidants: Vitamins A, E, and selenium are examples of antioxidants that help shield collagen from free radical-induced oxidative damage. Antioxidant-rich foods, such as leafy greens, berries, nuts, seeds, and colorful fruits and vegetables, can support young skin, the immune system, and general health by preserving the integrity of collagen.

Hyaluronic acid: The body naturally produces hyaluronic acid, which aids in preserving the hydration and suppleness of the skin. Collagen can help hydrate skin and maintain joint health when combined with foods high in hyaluronic acid, such as leafy greens, root vegetables, bone broth, and soy products.

Silica: A trace mineral, silica aids in the synthesis of collagen and preserves the suppleness and strength of connective tissues. Foods rich in silica, such cucumbers, brown rice, bananas, and oats, can maintain healthy skin, hair, and nails in addition to enhancing collagen supplements.

Gelatin: Derived from collagen, gelatin has comparable amino acids that aid in the manufacture of collagen and the repair of damaged tissue. Eating foods high in gelatin, such as homemade bone broth, desserts made with gelatin, and snacks created with collagen, can help promote intestinal integrity, skin rejuvenation, and joint health even more.

Zinc: An important mineral that is necessary for collagen formation, wound healing, and immune system function is zinc. When combined with collagen supplements, foods high in zinc, like shellfish, red meat, chicken, nuts, seeds, and legumes, can help promote the creation of collagen and aid in tissue healing.

Copper: Another trace mineral, copper plays a role in the production of collagen and in the cross-linking process that preserves the structural integrity of connective tissues. Collagen helps maintain healthy skin, hair, and joints. Copper-rich meals include organ meats, shellfish, nuts, seeds, and whole grains.

Magnesium: The body needs magnesium for hundreds of enzymatic processes, including those that produce collagen and maintain muscle tone. In addition to collagen supplements, foods high in magnesium, such as leafy greens, nuts, seeds, whole grains, and legumes, can promote general health and wellbeing.

Vitamin E: Vitamin E is a potent antioxidant that promotes skin health and wound healing while shielding collagen from oxidative damage. Combining collagen with foods high in vitamin E, such as nuts, seeds, avocado, spinach, and broccoli, helps support healthy skin, hair, and nails.

Sulfur: The production of collagen and the upkeep of strong connective tissues depend on the mineral sulfur. Garlic, onions, cruciferous vegetables, eggs, and other foods high in sulfur compounds can enhance the synthesis of collagen and improve the flexibility and health of joints.

Biotin: Also referred to as vitamin B7, biotin helps to produce keratin, which is necessary for healthy skin, hair, and nails. In addition to collagen, eating foods high in biotin, such as sweet potatoes, almonds, seeds, and eggs, can improve the general health of your skin and hair.

Vitamin K: This nutrient may be involved in the metabolism of collagen and is necessary for healthy bones and blood coagulation. When paired with collagen supplements, foods strong in vitamin K, such as leafy greens, broccoli, Brussels sprouts, and fermented foods, can promote collagen production and bone density.

Coenzyme Q10, or CoQ10, is a potent antioxidant that promotes energy synthesis in the mitochondria and shields cells from oxidative damage. Eating collagen-boosting foods high in CoQ10, such as nuts, whole grains, fatty fish, and organ meats, can also improve cardiovascular health and general vigor.

You may boost collagen's efficacy and support a number of health factors, such as bone density, skin elasticity, joint function, and general vitality, by mixing it with these extra nutrients. Including a variety of foods in your diet gives your body the fundamental building blocks it needs to grow and stay in maximum health.

CHAPTER 7

INVESTIGATING COLLAGEN SUPPLEMENTS

Collagen supplements are becoming a well-liked option in the field of health and wellbeing for boosting general vigor, improving joint function, and increasing skin health. Collagen is essential for preserving the integrity and structure of many different tissues, such as cartilage, skin, and bones. The natural collagen production in our bodies decreases with age, resulting in wrinkles, drooping skin, and sore joints. In order to maintain and increase collagen levels and promote optimum health and wellbeing, collagen supplements provide a practical and efficient solution.

When choosing a collagen supplement, one of the most important things to take into account is its bioavailability or how well the body absorbs and uses the collagen. Since smaller peptides are easier for the body to digest and absorb, collagen supplements that have undergone hydrolysis typically have higher bioavailability. The bioavailability of collagen may also be influenced by its source; marine collagen is frequently hailed for having a higher absorption rate than collagen from other sources.

Different Kinds of Collagen Supplements: Examining Choices for Ideal Health

There are many different kinds of collagen supplements, each with special advantages and obtained from diverse sources. People can select the collagen supplement that best meets their needs and preferences for health by being aware of the various types available. Here, we examine the most popular varieties of collagen supplements and their unique qualities:

Bovine Collagen: One of the most popular forms of collagen supplements comes from the skin, bones, and connective tissues of cows. Rich in type I and type III collagen, it helps to maintain general tissue integrity, bone strength, and skin elasticity. Hydroxylating bovine collagen increases its bioavailability, which facilitates absorption and utilization by the body.

Marine collagen: which comes from fish and other marine sources including shells and scales, is well known for having a high type I collagen concentration and good bioavailability. Because marine collagen peptides are smaller than bovine collagen peptides, the body can absorb them more readily. Marine collagen helps to hydrate skin, minimize wrinkles, and maintain joint health.

Porcine Collagen: The skin and connective tissues of pigs are the source of porcine collagen, which is similar to bovine collagen in terms of composition and health advantages. The potential of porcine collagen supplements to enhance tissue repair, improve skin suppleness, and aid in wound healing makes them popular in skincare products and wound dressings.

Chicken Collagen: Mostly made up of type II collagen, chicken collagen is collected from the skin, cartilage, and bones of chickens. Chicken collagen supplements are a popular option for people with arthritis or joint discomfort since type II collagen is particularly helpful for promoting joint health and mobility. Additionally thought to support skin suppleness and health is chicken collagen.

Multi-Collagen Blends: These blends offer a wide variety of collagen types by combining collagen from several sources, including chicken, eggshell, bovine, and marine collagen. The health of your skin, joints, bones, and digestive system are just a few of the many advantages that these mixtures provide. For those who want to use a single supplement to address several areas of their health, multi-collagen blends are great.

Collagen supplements provide a flexible and efficient means of promoting general health and wellness. People can maximize their health and vitality by choosing collagen supplements wisely and by being aware of the various kinds available as well as their distinct qualities.

Types of collagen supplements:

1. **Collagen Peptides:** One of the most well-liked types of collagen supplements is collagen peptides, sometimes referred to as hydrolyzed collagen or collagen hydrolysate. Usually, they come from animal collagen such fish skin, chicken sternum, or cow hide. The process of converting collagen molecules into smaller peptides, which the body can absorb and use more easily, is known as collagen peptide processing. They are adaptable and simple to add to a variety of drinks and meals because they frequently have no flavor or smell.

2. **Collagen Powder:** Another popular type of collagen supplement is collagen powder. Usually composed of collagen peptides, they are simple to incorporate into drinks like smoothies, juice, or water. There are many flavors available for collagen powders, including unflavored, flavored, and flavored with extra components like antioxidants, vitamins, or minerals.

3. **Collagen Capsules**: Collagen peptides and powders can be packaged in in a vegetarian or gelatin capsule. They are perfect for people who dislike the texture or flavor of collagen powders and would rather have the ease of a pre-measured dosage.

4. **Liquid Collage:** You can drink liquid collagen supplements straight or mix them with juice or water. Colloidal supplements come in a liquid form. The usual recipe for these is to dissolve collagen peptides in water or a flavor-infused liquid base. For those who would rather take collagen supplements on the go in a quick and simple manner, liquid collagen supplements are a great option.

5. **Collagen Gummies:** For individuals who would rather take their collagen in a more pleasurable method, collagen gummies are a sweet and

practical choice. To make chewy and tasty gummy supplements, collagen peptides, fruit juice, and sweeteners are mixed together. Collagen gummies come in a variety of tastes and are frequently enhanced with vitamins and minerals to provide even more health advantages.

6. **Collagen Bars:** Packed with various components including almonds, seeds, and dried fruits, collagen bars are a portable and easy-to-carry snack that contains collagen peptides. They are perfect for anyone who want to increase their intake of collagen while on the road in a quick and nourishing method. Collagen bars are available in a range of tastes and are frequently low in sugar and gluten.

7. **Collagen Creams and Lotions:** Topical skincare products that contain collagen peptides or substances that promote collagen are known as collagen creams and lotions. They aid to increase the moisture, elasticity, and firmness of the skin when applied directly to the skin. To improve the general health and appearance of the skin, oral collagen supplements are frequently used with collagen creams and lotions.

These represent some of the most popular collagen supplement varieties on the market. Every variant presents distinct advantages and benefits, enabling people to select the one that most closely aligns with their interests and way of life.

CHAPTER 8

COLLAGEN DIET/ SUPPLEMENTATION FOR SPECIFIC HEALTH GOALS

We have covered the foundations of the collagen diet in earlier chapters, along with tips for optimizing its advantages and sources. Let us now explore how the collagen diet can be customized to target particular health objectives and issues. You may tailor the collagen diet to your specific goals, whether they be to control weight, improve joint function, maintain skin health, or improve sports performance.

We will look at applying the collagen diet's tenets to particular health goals in this chapter. With the backing of scientific research and useful insights, we will offer specific advice and meal plans that promote different health objectives. The collagen diet provides adaptable options to meet your specific goals, whether you want to improve overall well-being, reduce joint discomfort, increase energy, or regenerate your skin.

You will be able to design a customized nutrition plan that supports your objectives and make educated food decisions by knowing how collagen and particular nutrients work with the body to support various elements of health. The collagen diet can be an effective tool for reaching your goals, whether you are trying to lose weight, healing from an injury, or just wanting to improve your overall health and energy.

Let us investigate how you might use the collagen diet to reach your individual health objectives and realize your greatest potential in terms of life, health, and energy. Whether your goal is to strengthen your joints, improve your complexion, become more athletic, or reach a healthy weight, the collagen diet provides an adaptable and efficient method that you can customize to your own requirements and tastes. Together, let us take this trip to uncover the collagen diet's transformative power and help you reach your wellness and health goals.

The Collagen Diet: A Weight Loss Plan

We shall look at how to modify the collagen diet to help achieve weight loss objectives in this part. We will talk about how collagen supports overall metabolic health, increases satiety, and speeds up metabolism.

Encouraging Satiety: High in satiating protein, collagen can aid in lowering cravings and hunger, which will make it simpler to stick to a diet low in calories. Incorporating collagen-rich foods like bone broth, lean meats, chicken, fish, eggs, and dairy products into meals and snacks might help decrease overall calorie intake by promoting feelings of fullness and satisfaction.

Maintaining Lean Muscle Mass: Maintaining lean muscle mass is crucial for maintaining metabolic health and preventing muscle loss when trying to lose weight. Essential amino acids included in collagen are necessary for both muscle growth and repair. Eating foods high in collagen along with other sources of premium protein can support a healthy body composition and assist preserve muscle mass while losing weight.

Increasing Metabolism: Research has indicated that collagen promotes energy expenditure and supports metabolic processes, both of which can aid in weight loss. You may boost your weight reduction efforts by increasing your metabolic rate and promoting fat burning by incorporating collagen supplements or foods high in collagen into your diet.

Improving Gut Health: For the best possible metabolism, nutrition absorption, and digestion, a healthy gut microbiota is necessary. Amino acids included in collagen, such as glutamine and glycine, boost gut health, may lessen inflammation, and enhance digestive function. Consuming collagen-rich foods and supplements, such as bone broth, can improve intestinal integrity and encourage maintaining a healthy weight.

Stabilizing Blood Sugar: Studies have demonstrated that collagen peptides enhance insulin sensitivity and control blood sugar, which can help ward off cravings and encourage consistent energy levels all day. Eating complex carbs, high-fiber meals, and healthy fats with collagen can help stabilize blood sugar levels and lower the chance of overindulging.

You can improve your nutrition to encourage fat reduction, preserve lean muscle mass, and achieve long-lasting outcomes by combining foods high in collagen, collagen supplements, and focused dietary techniques into your weight loss plan. A balanced diet, drinking plenty of water, exercising frequently, and controlling stress are other crucial elements of a successful weight loss program. In addition to helping you lose weight, the collagen diet can also help you improve your general health and well-being if you follow it with commitment, consistency, and a customized strategy.

Collagen Supplementation for Bone Health:

We shall look at collagen's function in supporting joint health and reducing symptoms associated with joints in this section. We will highlight how collagen enhances joint flexibility and mobility, lowers inflammation and discomfort, and supports the integrity and structure of joint cartilage.

Underpinning Joint Structure: Collagen is the main building block of joint cartilage, the connective tissue that cushions and shields the ends of bones within joints. The body's natural production of collagen decreases with age, which increases the risk of joint-related problems like osteoarthritis and causes cartilage to break down. Collagen peptide supplements can enhance the general health of joints by supporting the structural integrity of joint cartilage.

Enhancing Joint Flexibility and Mobility: Research has demonstrated that using collagen supplements can enhance joint flexibility and mobility, which will make it simpler to carry out daily tasks and engage in physical activity. Collagen helps people move more freely and pleasantly by improving joint lubrication and lowering friction between joint surfaces, which helps relieve stiffness and discomfort brought on by diseases like rheumatoid arthritis and osteoarthritis.

Mitigating Inflammation and Pain: Prolonged inflammation is frequently the root cause of various joint-related ailments, leading to discomfort, edema, and tissue impairment. Anti-inflammatory substances like proline and glycine found in collagen can help relieve joint discomfort and inflammation. It may be possible to maintain a healthy inflammatory response and increase joint comfort and mobility by including collagen supplements or foods high in collagen in your diet.

Supporting Tendon and Ligament Health: Collagen is critical for maintaining the structure and function of tendons and ligaments, which are necessary for joint stability and movement, in addition to supporting the health of joint cartilage. Collagen peptide supplements can decrease the chance of injury, improve general joint stability and function, and strengthen tendons and ligaments.

Improving Recuperation and Repair: Research has demonstrated that collagen supplements can hasten the healing process after joint replacements or accidents by encouraging tissue regeneration and repair. Collagen supplements provide the building blocks needed for collagen production, which can speed up healing, lessen recovery time, and enhance overall results.

Including a collagen supplement in your daily regimen can help promote joint health, reduce discomfort, and preserve flexibility and mobility as you age. A thorough joint health program also includes adopting a balanced diet full of nutrient-dense foods, drinking plenty of water, exercising frequently, and using stress-reduction strategies. Collagen supplementation is a safe, all-natural way to promote joint health and improve overall quality of life because of its many advantages and few adverse effects.

Gut Health with Collagen:

We shall look at collagen's function in preserving gut health and resolving digestive problems in this section. We will review how collagen supports a balanced gut flora, supports healthy digestion, and maintains the integrity of the gut lining.

Maintaining the Integrity of the Gut Lining: The gut lining acts as a barrier to keep the body safe from noxious things including infections, poisons, and leftover food particles. Amino acids such as glutamine and glycine found in collagen are critical for supporting gut barrier function and preserving the integrity of the intestinal lining. Collagen peptide supplements can lessen intestinal permeability, or "leaky gut," reinforce the gut lining, and guard against immunological and digestive disorders.

Encouraging Digestive Health: Gelatin, a component of collagen, coats the digestive track and makes it easier for food to pass through the stomach. Eating foods high in collagen, such as bone broth, or taking collagen supplements can improve regular bowel movements, ease indigestion, and support good digestion. Furthermore, collagen's capacity to protect the mucosal lining of the gut may aid in lowering inflammation and enhancing general digestive health.

Gut Microbiome Balance: The population of bacteria that live in the digestive tract, also known as the gut microbiome, is essential for immune system response, metabolism, and digestive health. Studies have demonstrated that taking supplements of collagen can help maintain a healthy gut microbiome by having prebiotic-like actions that encourage the development of good bacteria. Collagen can sustain gut health and promote general well-being by fostering a varied and balanced gut microbiota.

Reducing Inflammation: Irritable bowel syndrome (IBS), inflammatory bowel disease (IBD), and leaky gut syndrome are among the digestive illnesses linked to chronic inflammation in the gut. Anti-inflammatory substances included in collagen can help lessen intestinal lining inflammation and ease the symptoms of digestive pain. Including collagen-rich foods or supplements in your diet may assist to support a normal inflammatory response and encourage the healing of your gut.

Collagen Supplementation: Research indicates that collagen supplements can aid in the healing of the gut by mending damaged intestinal tissues. Collagen supplements provide the building blocks needed for collagen production, which might hasten healing after inflammatory flare-ups, infections, or injuries to the gastrointestinal tract. Furthermore, collagen's capacity to maintain the integrity of the gut lining may aid in halting additional harm and advancing long-term intestinal health. Including a collagen supplement in your daily regimen can help improve gut health, ease digestive problems, and enhance general wellbeing. A thorough gut health program also includes eating a balanced diet high in fiber, foods high in probiotics, and foods that are high in nutrients, drinking plenty of water, controlling stress, and engaging in regular exercise. Collagen supplementation offers a safe and natural way to promote gut health and improve overall digestive function, with many advantages and few adverse effects.

A Collagen Diet for Healthy Skin:

We shall look at collagen's function in boosting skin health and vibrancy in this section. We will see how collagen stimulates the production of new collagen, maintains the skin's structure and function, and guards against the effects of aging.

Supporting Skin Structure: Collagen gives the skin its elasticity, firmness, and strength. The body's natural production of collagen decreases with age, causing drooping, wrinkles, and a loss of suppleness. Collagen peptide supplements can help maintain the skin's structural integrity, which will help to smooth out fine lines and wrinkles and provide the appearance of younger skin.

Encouraging Collagen Synthesis: Research has demonstrated that collagen supplements can enhance the skin's synthesis of collagen, resulting in enhanced hydration, suppleness, and texture. Collagen supplements can help restore lost collagen and encourage skin cell renewal by giving the building blocks needed for collagen creation. This will give the look of a more youthful and vibrant skin.

Improving Skin Hydration: By trapping moisture in the skin's layers, collagen is essential for preserving skin hydration. Collagen peptide supplements can help hydrate the skin more deeply, which will lessen flakiness, roughness, and dryness. Collagen also aids in the synthesis of hyaluronic acid, a chemical that retains water in the skin and increases its plumpness and moisture.

Preventing UV Damage: Antioxidant qualities found in collagen aid in shielding the skin from UV rays and oxidative stress. Collagen supplements can help avoid sun-induced premature aging, which includes sunspots, fine lines, and wrinkles, by scavenging free radicals and lowering inflammation. Nevertheless, for the best possible skin protection, utilize collagen supplements along with sunscreen and sun safety precautions.

Collagen is essential for supporting wound healing because it stimulates tissue regeneration and repair. Collagen peptide supplements can hasten the healing of cuts, wounds, and abrasions, minimizing scarring and encouraging a quicker recovery. Collagen also aids in the development of new blood vessels, which facilitates the delivery of nutrients and oxygen to the skin and speeds up the healing process.

A Collagen Diet for Healthy Hair and Nails:

We shall discuss collagen's involvement in fostering healthy hair and nails in this section. We will talk about how collagen helps to prevent damage and breakage, encourages growth and thickness, and supports the structure of hair and nails.

Strengthening and Supporting Hair Structure: Collagen is an essential part of the hair follicle that gives it strength and support. Collagen peptide supplements can thicken the hair shaft, lessen breakage, and encourage strong, healthy growth. Collagen also aids in the synthesis of keratin, a protein that is found in most hair strands improving the strength and durability of hair,

Enhancing Hair Growth: Research has demonstrated that taking collagen supplements can enhance hair follicle activity and augment hair growth. Collagen promotes the growth phase of the hair cycle by giving vital amino acids and nutrients, which over time results in thicker, fuller hair. Collagen also enhances scalp blood circulation, which supplies nutrients and oxygen to hair follicles and encourages healthy hair growth.

Increasing Nail Strength: A significant part of the nail matrix, which is the tissue underlying the nail bed and is responsible for nail growth and strength, is collagen. Collagen peptide supplements can improve the strength of the nail matrix and lessen breakage, splitting, and brittleness. Collagen also helps the nails produce more keratin, which increases the strength and durability of the nails.

Encouraging Nail Growth: Research indicates that taking a collagen supplement helps encourage nail growth by giving the body the vital nutrients required for nail development and repair. Collagen promotes the growth of longer, stronger, and healthier nails by promoting the division of nail cells and improving circulation in the nail bed. Collagen also helps the nails retain moisture, which lessens dryness and increases suppleness.

Preventing Breakage and Damage: Supplementing with collagen helps shield hair and nails from breakage and damage brought on by chemicals, styling tools, and harsh environmental conditions. Collagen makes hair and nails more structurally sound, which lessens the chance of breakage, split ends, and brittleness. Collagen also helps hair and nails retain moisture better, which reduces dryness and increases general resilience.

Including collagen supplements in your daily regimen can help maintain the health of your hair and nails, encourage growth, and guard against breakage and damage.

CHAPTER 9

BONE BROTH PREPARATION

For many years, people have valued bone broth as a richly flavorful, nourishing elixir. High bioavailable collagen content is one of its most sought-after qualities. This important protein promotes skin, joint, and gut health among other areas of wellness. We look at the skill of creating bone broth in this chapter as well as how to use its collagen content for maximum health and energy.

Knowing Collagen and Bone Broth

Long-simmered bones, connective tissues, and aromatics in water yields a nutrient-dense liquid called bone broth. A tasty and nutrient-dense elixir is produced as the bones simmer and release collagen, gelatin, minerals, and other nutrients into the broth.

Bone Broth Preparation

Start with premium bones from pastured chicken, wild-caught fish, or cattle reared on grass. Fill a big pot or slow cooker halfway full of water with the bones. Add a little vinegar, such apple cider vinegar to aid in the bones' mineral extraction. Bring to boil, turn down heat to low and simmer the broth for at least 12 to 24 hours, preferably longer for the best flavor and nutrient extraction. Every now and again when cooking, skim off any foam or contaminants that rise to the top.

Increasing Collagen Content

To get the most collagen concentration in your bone broth, include fish heads and tails, cattle knuckles, or chicken feet. Collagen and gelatin abound in these sections, giving the soup even more richness and flavor. To improve the broth's flavor profile, add aromatic vegetables and herbs such onions, carrots, celery, garlic, and parsley.

Added Simmering Time:

Even though bone broth should simmer for at least 12 to 24 hours, boiling it longer can help to extract more collagen. For the broth to completely breakdown the collagen and release its nutrients, boil it for at least 48 hours. Higher collagen content and a richer, more delicious broth will come from this longer boiling time.

Reactive Media:

A lemon juice or apple cider vinegar addition to the bone broth can aid in the extraction of nutrients and collagen from the bones. The acid facilitates the improved absorption of nutrients into the soup by breaking down the collagen strands. Making bone broth, aim to add one to two tablespoons of vinegar or lemon juice every gallon of water.

Easy Heat:

The integrity of the collagen and other nutrients in the soup depends on keeping the simmering temperature low and steady. Thoroughly heating the soup can denature the proteins and make it less collagen-rich. Rather, let the soup simmer slowly over low heat so that its flavors gradually come through.

You can optimize the collagen content of your bone broth and be sure you are getting the most out of this nutritious elixir by using these methods and advice. To achieve the ideal ratio of flavor to nutrient density in your own bone broth, play about with various ingredients, simmering times, and cooking techniques.

Collagen from Bone Broth

Once prepared, your bone broth can be used as a foundation for soups, stews, sauces, and other dishes or enjoyed as a warm and healthy drink on its own. Because bone broth contains a lot of collagen, drinking it on a regular basis can help maintain healthy skin, joints and digestion. It may also be used as an electrolyte replenishment and muscle development and repair drink after an exercise.

Making Bone Broth a Part of Your Regular Schedule

A cup of warm bone broth can be taken as a mid-morning or afternoon pick-me-up or as the foundation for homemade soups and stews. As a tasty cooking liquid for grains, beans, and vegetables, you can also drink bone broth before meals to aid in digestion.

With so many vitamins, minerals, and amino acids, bone broth is a nutrient-dense elixir with many health advantages. Learn how to prepare and use bone broth in your daily life to benefit from its collagen-rich richness for general health, radiant skin, and robust health. Get bone broth into your regimen and enjoy its nourishing qualities.

CHAPTER 10

TROUBLESHOOTING AND FAQS

There are a lot of questions, difficulties, and doubts you could have when you first start the collagen diet. We will go over common problems and often asked questions in this chapter so you can approach your collagen diet experience with assurance and clarity.

Here are the best responses to frequently asked questions concerning the collagen diet:

1. What daily amount of collagen should I take to get the best results?

Each person has different demands and objectives when it comes to collagen dosage recommendations. For healthy skin, hair, and nails, a daily dosage of 5–10 grams of hydrolyzed collagen or collagen peptides is usual. Higher doses (10–20 grams daily) may be helpful for joint health.

2. If I have dietary limitations or food allergies, can I still eat collagen?

Most collagen supplements come from animal sources, including marine or cow collagen. On the other hand, plant-based collagen substitutes are also available. Examples of these include collagen-boosting supplements that contain vitamins, minerals, and amino acids to assist the synthesis of collagen.

3. Do collagen supplements have any possible negative effects or interactions with medications?

For the majority of people, collagen supplements are safe when used as prescribed. Still, it is always a good idea to speak with a doctor, particularly if you are expecting, nursing, or taking medication, to make sure there are not any possible conflicts or side effects.

4. Which collagen-rich foods are the healthiest for vegans or vegetarians?

Consuming plant-based meals high in antioxidants, vitamin C, and amino acids—such as fruits, vegetables, nuts, seeds, legumes, and soy products—can help vegetarians and vegans increase the production of collagen. Furthermore, plant-based components like vitamin C, hyaluronic acid, and amino acids found in collagen-boosting supplements can aid in the manufacturing of collagen.

5. How long does collagen supplementation take to show results?

Collagen supplements outcomes can differ based on personal aspects like age, nutritional status, way of life, and general health. While some people may observe considerable benefits in skin elasticity, moisture, and texture within a few weeks of supplementing consistently, joint health and hair development may take several months to show major improvements.

6. Can supplements containing collagen help with particular skin disorders like eczema or acne?

Although they are not a panacea, collagen supplements may help lessen the symptoms of some skin problems and enhance the general health of the skin. In order to achieve the best results with collagen supplements for specific skin conditions like acne or eczema, it is critical to address underlying aspects like nutrition, skincare routine, and lifestyle behaviors.

7. Are women who are expecting or nursing safe to take collagen supplements?

Although most people find collagen supplements safe, women who are pregnant or nursing should speak with their healthcare professional before beginning any new supplement regimen to be sure it is safe and effective and to address any possible interactions or concerns.

8. Can taking collagen supplements aid in developing muscle

mass or losing weight?
By encouraging satiety, boosting metabolism, and maintaining lean muscle mass, collagen supplements may help weight loss and muscle growth in an indirect manner. Rather than being a stand-alone treatment for weight loss or muscle building, they ought to be a part of a well-rounded diet and exercise program.

9. Do other skincare treatments or products interact with collagen supplements?
It is possible to combine collagen supplements with other skincare products and treatments, as they are generally well tolerated. To avoid irritation or unfavorable consequences, it is crucial to adhere to skincare professionals' guidelines and refrain from overusing or layering products excessively.

10. Which collagen hydrolysate, collagen peptides, and gelatin is best for me? What are the distinctions between them?
Collagen protein is the source of collagen peptides, collagen hydrolysate, and gelatin; however, its bioavailability and processing methods vary. Collagen peptides are short chains of amino acids extracted through enzymatic hydrolysis. They are easier to absorb and are frequently chosen for their ease and adaptability. Gelation is a larger protein derived from collagen to produce a gel-like consistency that is ideal for use in recipes and other culinary applications. Collagen Hydrolysate is obtained from further processing of collagen into smaller peptides and amino acids, making it easier to absorb and digest in supplements, food and cosmetics. The ideal choice will vary depending on personal tastes and intended application.

11. Can supplements made of collagen take the place of a well-balanced diet?
Complete meals should always be the primary source of nourishment, even though collagen supplements can be a useful adjunct to a healthy diet. To satisfy your body's completely nutritional requirements, you must eat a range of nutrient-rich meals.

12. Are children able to take collagen supplements?

Although collagen supplements are typically safe for kids, it is best to check with a pediatrician to be sure your child's age and developmental stage are suitable before giving them collagen supplements.

13. Is it possible to reduce cellulite with collagen supplements?

Though there is little scientific proof to support collagen supplements' ability to specifically reduce cellulite, studies have shown that collagen may increase skin firmness and elasticity. For reducing cellulite, a healthy lifestyle that includes regular exercise and a balanced diet may be more beneficial.

14. Do collagen supplements smell or taste like anything?

Since collagen supplements usually have no taste or smell, it is simple to add them to a variety of foods and drinks without changing their flavor or aroma. However, depending on the brand and formulation, some people can detect a faint taste or odor.

15. Can taking collagen supplements aid in thinning or hair loss?

Collagen supplements can help hair grow and stay healthy by giving the scalp the necessary nutrients and encouraging the production of collagen. Used in conjunction with other hair care practices and treatments, they may help improve overall hair quality but are not a cure for thinning or hair loss.

16. Are collagen supplements safe for diabetics to take?

For those with diabetes, collagen supplements are generally safe, but it is important to regularly check blood sugar levels, particularly if taking large amounts or combining them with other supplements. Before beginning collagen supplementation, see a doctor if you have diabetes or any other medical problem.

17. Can supplements containing collagen assist with arthritis and joint pain?

Research has demonstrated that taking collagen supplements can improve joint health by supplying vital nutrients for cartilage restoration and lowering joint inflammation. While some people may find that they assist in reducing the symptoms of arthritis and joint pain, the effects might vary, so it is important to speak with a healthcare professional for specific advice.

18. Are there any age limits on collagen supplements?

For adults of all ages, collagen supplements are typically safe, but it is important to adhere to suggested amounts and see a doctor, particularly for older folks or those with underlying medical concerns.

19. Can collagen supplements aid in the healing process after a workout?

Because they supply necessary amino acids for muscle repair and encourage the production of collagen in connective tissues, collagen supplements may aid in the recovery process following an exercise. Taking collagen supplements with a well-balanced post-workout meal or smoothie can improve muscle repair and recuperation.

20. What is the best way to keep collagen supplements so they stay fresh?

For optimal freshness and effectiveness, store collagen supplements in a cool, dry location away from moisture and direct sunlight. The quality of collagen supplements might deteriorate with time, so keep them away from heat sources and humid surroundings.

Modifications for Dietary Restrictions (such as Dairy-Free and Gluten-Free):

Gluten-Free:

To make sure they do not have any gluten-containing ingredients, look for collagen supplements that have received the gluten-free certification. Choose gluten-free collagen powders or capsules, and carefully study ingredient labels to be certain of any possible gluten sources.
Lean meats, chicken, fish, eggs, fruits, vegetables, nuts, seeds, and gluten-free grains like quinoa, rice, and buckwheat are among the naturally gluten-free, collagen-rich foods to choose.

Non-dairy:
If dairy is an issue for you, look for collagen supplements that come from
plant- or marine-based sources, including collagen from fruits and
vegetables or marine collagen.
Stay away from collagen supplements that have ingredients derived from
dairy, such as milk powder or whey protein. Choose hydrolyzed collagen or
pure collagen peptides without any additional dairy ingredients.
Include dairy-free collagen sources in your diet, such as fish or poultry
bones used to make bone broth, or foods high in collagen, such as leafy
greens, berries, citrus fruits, and soy products.

Vegan or vegetarian?
To promote collagen production without using substances sourced from
animals, go for plant-based collagen substitutes that include nutrients like
vitamin C, amino acids, and antioxidants.
Seek for collagen-enhancing supplements derived from plant-based sources
including antioxidant-rich herbs (like rosehip, green tea), vitamin C-rich
fruits (like acerola cherries), and legumes (like beans, lentils) that are high
in amino acids.
To stimulate natural collagen production, include foods high in protein,
including legumes and pulses, vitamin C-rich fruits and vegetables, and
antioxidant-rich nuts and seeds, in your diet.

Allergies to nuts:
To prevent any potential adverse reactions, look for collagen supplements
devoid of common allergens including almonds and tree nuts.
Select collagen supplements that come from production facilities with
specialized techniques to prevent cross-contamination with nuts and other
allergens, as well as rigorous adherence to allergen control procedures.
Choose pure collagen peptides or hydrolyzed collagen without any
additional nut ingredients when choosing collagen supplements. Stay clear
of supplements that contain flavors or additives derived from nuts, such as
almond extract or coconut milk powder.

Free of Soy:
To prevent any allergic reactions or sensitivities, choose collagen supplements free of soy-based chemicals or fillers, such as soy lecithin or soy protein isolate.
To make sure collagen supplements do not contain any soy-derived substances, carefully study ingredient labels and look for supplements that are specifically labelled as soy-free.
Select foods high in collagen and nutrients that increase collagen from non-soy sources, such as fish, poultry, lean meats, fruits, vegetables, nuts, and seeds; alternate sources of protein include pea protein and hemp protein.

APPENDIX: GLOSSARY OF TERMS

Collagen: This structural protein is present in the skin, hair, nails, and connective tissues of the body. It gives these tissues stability, flexibility, and strength.

Peptides of Collagen: Collagen peptides, often referred to as collagen hydrolysate or collagen hydrolysate, are smaller, more readily absorbed versions of animal collagen that have undergone hydrolysis. To promote better absorption, they are frequently used in collagen supplements.

Hydrolyzed Collagen: This is a procedure whereby hydrolysis breaks down collagen into smaller peptides of collagen. The body can absorb and use this type of collagen more easily.

Collagen Synthesis: The process by which the body creates new collagen molecules. Age, genetics, food, and general health all have an impact on collagen synthesis.

Marine Collagen: This is collagen obtained from the deep e.g., collagen obtained from the skin and scales of fish through a process of hydroxylation.

Amino acids: The building blocks of all proteins, including collagen. Amino acids are vital for the formation of collagen and are important for preserving general health and wellbeing.

Antioxidants: These substances aid in shielding the body from the damaging effects of free radicals and oxidative stress. Numerous foods, such as fruits, vegetables, nuts, and seeds, contain antioxidants, which are crucial for maintaining healthy skin and preventing aging.

Hyaluronic acid: The body naturally produces hyaluronic acid, which aids in preserving the hydration and lubrication of the skin. Hyaluronic acid's hydrating and anti-aging qualities make it a popular ingredient in skincare products and supplements.

Vitamin C is a necessary nutrient that is important for the formation of collagen. Numerous fruits and vegetables, including bell peppers, oranges, strawberries, and kiwis, are good sources of vitamin C.

Elastin: An additional protein type that gives elasticity and resilience, it is present in the skin and connective tissues. Collagen and elastin work together to maintain the structure and functionality of the skin.

Free Radicals: Unstable chemicals that can lead to oxidative stress, which damages tissues and cells. Pollution, UV radiation, and bad lifestyle choices are some of the things that produce free radicals, which can hasten aging and disease.

Inflammation: Redness, swelling, pain, and heat are the body's normal reactions to injury, infection, or irritation. Chronic inflammation is a factor in many health concerns, such as joint discomfort and skin disorders.

Oxidative stress: This is the outcome of an imbalance that occurs between the body's generation of free radicals and its antioxidant capacity, which leads to cellular damage. Ageing, illness, and skin problems are associated with oxidative stress.

Skin Elasticity: The skin's capacity to expand and contract in reaction to pressure or movement. The suppleness of the skin, which keeps the skin smooth, firm, and youthful-looking, is greatly dependent on collagen.

UV Radiation: The sun's ultraviolet rays can permeate the skin and harm it, leading to accelerated aging, sunburns, and skin cancer. Keeping the skin healthy requires protecting it from UV rays.

Wrinkles: The creases, folds, or lines that appear in the skin due to aging, sun exposure, and other causes. Wrinkles are a result of a reduction in skin suppleness and collagen production.

Bone Density: A measurement of the mineral content in bone tissue that reveals the density and strength of the bone. By offering vital nutrients for bone growth and repair, collagen supplements may promote bone health and density.

Joint mobility: This is the capacity of joints to move through their whole range of motion with ease and without restriction. Cartilage is the tissue that surrounds and cushions joints, allowing for flexibility and motion. One of its main ingredients is collagen.

The aging process: This is the normal biological process of becoming older, marked by modifications to the structure, functionality, and appearance of the body. Visible indicators of aging, such wrinkles, drooping skin, and stiff joints, are caused by a decrease in collagen synthesis and a loss of collagen.

REFERENCES

Borumand, M., & Sibilla, S. (2014). Daily consumption of the collagen supplement Pure Gold Collagen® reduces visible signs of aging. Clinical Interventions in Aging, 9, 1747–1758.

Hexsel, D., Zague, V., Schunck, M., Siega, C., & Camozzato, F. O. (2017). Oral supplementation with specific bioactive collagen peptides improves nail growth and reduces symptoms of brittle nails. Journal of Cosmetic Dermatology, 16(4), 520–526.

Zdzieblik, D., Oesser, S., Gollhofer, A., & König, D. (2015). Improvement of activity-related knee joint discomfort following supplementation of specific collagen peptides. Applied Physiology, Nutrition, and Metabolism, 42(6), 588–595.

Proksch E, Segger D, Degwert J, Schunck M, Zague V, Oesser S. Oral supplementation of specific collagen peptides has beneficial effects on human skin physiology: a double-blind, placebo-controlled study. Skin Pharmacol Physiol. 2014; 27(1):47-55. Doe: 10.1159/000351376

Asserin J, Lati E, Shioya T, Prawitt J. The effect of oral collagen peptide supplementation on skin moisture and the dermal collagen network: evidence from an ex vivo model and randomized, placebo-controlled clinical trials. J Cosmet Dermatol. 2015; 14(4):291-301. doi:10.1111/jocd.12174

Borumand M, Sibilla S. Daily consumption of the collagen supplement Pure Gold Collagen® reduces visible signs of aging. Clin Interv Aging. 2014; 9:1747-1758. doi:10.2147/CIA.S65939